A. Mostafawy

Pediatric Sonoencephalography

The Practical Use of Ultrasonic Echoes
in the Diagnosis of Childhood Intracranial Disorders

In Cooperation with J. B. Nagle

With 52 Figures

Springer-Verlag Berlin · Heidelberg · New York 1971

Dr. ABBAS MOSTAFAWY, Universitäts-Kinderklinik, 6900 Heidelberg, Germany

ISBN-13: 978-3-642-65088-8 e-ISBN-13: 978-3-642-65086-4
DOI: 10.1007/978-3-642-65086-4

Softcover reprint of the hardcover 1st edition 1971
 Typesetting, printing and binding: Konrad Triltsch, Graphischer Betrieb, 87 Würzburg, Germany.

Foreword

Clinical sono-encephalography, although a relatively new technique, is rapidly gaining acceptance in hospital and specialist practice. No problem was involved in its introduction, as the method is self-evidently suitable for the diagnosis of acute and chronic intracranial lesions. As an auxiliary examination it is, within its limitations, almost ideal: it requires no large investment in apparatus, it is rapidly done, the patient suffers no discomfort, and there is no risk of complications. In the hands of an experienced examiner, who has a solid grounding in neurological theory and practice to enable him to interpret his findings, it yields important and reliable information.

The use of this method in children requires special knowledge, covering the age of the child, the technique of examination, the range of normality and the interpretation of the pathological findings from the neuropediatric point of view. These special features of pediatric sono-encephalography are seldom discussed in the literature, wide as it is. This monograph is designed to bridge the gap.

The book is based on the author's extensive experience acquired over a number of years in the neuropediatric department of the University Children's Hospital Heidelberg. Wisely used, pediatric sono-encephalography should provide a useful tool, not only for experts in highly specialized hospital departments, but also for pediatricians, neuropediatricians, child psychiatrists, neurologists and neurosurgeons engaged in more routine clinical work.

Heidelberg, February 1971 HORST BICKEL

Preface

Neuropediatrics has experienced enormous advances within recent years. New diagnostic examination procedures have contributed considerably to these advances. Aside from such conventional procedures as pneumoencephalography and electroencephalography, one should also mention cerebral angiography, brain scintiscanning and, in a special sense, sonoencephalography.

Sonoencephalographic examination of adult subjects has received considerable attention, especially in such monographs as those published by GROSSMAN, SCHIEFER and KAZNER, and PIA and GELETNEKY. To date, a basic presentation of the sonoencephalographic examination in children does not exist. Consequently, I have attempted to compile a work covering the entire spectrum of the sonoencephalographic examination in pediatrics. For this purpose I have had at my disposal the observations and information gained from 1500 patients and more than 4500 sonoencephalograms. A large portion of these examinations has been substantiated by pneumoencephalography, electroencephalography, and angiography. Valuable diagnostic assistance could be contributed by the sonoencephalogram in the general neurological evaluation of the child. Its particular advantages are that it is accurate, convenient, rapid, harmless, and painless for the patient and can be repeated as often as desired. When sonoencephalographic results are combined with those obtained from the electroencephalogram, the diagnostic possibilities of each are enhanced. In association with the neurology department at the University of Heidelberg Children's Hospital, valuable experiences could be obtained in all areas of neuropediatrics. In particular, it has been possible to comprehensively study such areas as brain damage during early childhood, cerebral damage resulting from inborn errors of metabolism, CNS congenital defects, and convulsive disorders.

At this point I would like to express my indebtedness especially to Dr. R. KRUSE, former director of the department of neurology, University of Heidelberg Children's Hospital, and present director of the Korker Anstalten, Kork, W. Germany. Dr. KRUSE's cooperation and the noble support of the Director of the Children's Hospital of the University of Heidelberg, my highly respected Professor H. BICKEL, enabled me to found the department of sonoencephalography at the Children's Hospital and to develop it to its present capacity. My particular thanks go also to my colleagues of the sonoencephalographic department: G. VON CZETTRITZ, K. WINTER, and D. MEYER. I thank, too, my doctoral candidate, J. B. NAGLE, for his many and varied efforts; he also prepared the translation.

I would like to express my sincere appreciation to Dr. SCHEFFNER, present director of the neurology department of the University of Heidelberg Children's Hospital, and his assistants, as well as to Dr. WILLICH, director of the roentgenology department, and his staff for their active assistance and advice. I owe considerable thanks to Prof. Dr. PENZHOLZ, director of the neurosurgery department of the University of Heidelberg Surgical Hospital, and Dr. PISCOL for providing angiograms and medical records. I received generous co-operation from Karl Müller & Co., Heidelberg, who graciously donated the ultrasonic apparatus by Kretz-Technik through their Managing Director in West Germany, Mr. BELUT, Heppenheim. I am also grateful for the valuable technical assistance so generously given by Siemens Electronics in Mannheim. Special credit goes to draftsman J. SCHNEIDER for his vividly expressed schematic illustrations. Grateful acknowledgment goes to Mr. WISMAC for his valuable mathematical computations and to the Computer Center of the University of Heidelberg. Special thanks goes to Mrs. SUSAN TUTTLE for helping with the proof reading and to Mrs. ELISABETH MORGNER for relinquishing valuable secretarial assistance. Most special thanks goes to Miss PATRICIA BOEHLEN for assisting in preparation of this text.

I would also like to express my sincere appreciation to the Springer-Verlag for its generous co-operation and understanding concessions.

Heidelberg, July 1970 A. MOSTAFAWY

Contents

Introduction 1

Part One: General Sonoencephalography

Chapter I General Physical Properties of Sound in Liquids and Gases . . 2
A. Classification of Sounds 4
B. Physical Characteristics of Ultrasound 4
C. Laws of Reflection and Refraction 4
D. Conditions Favorable to Reflection 5
E. Diffraction 6
F. Sound Scattering and Absorption (Sound Attenuation) . . 6

Chapter II Technical Considerations of the Ultrasonic Impulse Apparatus . 7
A. Construction of the A-scope Apparatus 7
1. Transmitter 8
2. Sound Receiver 9
3.—5. The Screen Image (Synchronization Unit, Indicator Gauge, and Sweep Generator) 10
B. Linear-Scanning 12
C.—E. Arc-, Sector- and Compound-Scanning 13

Chapter III Examination of Pediatric Patient 13
A. Examination Procedure with Patient in the Supine Position 13
B. Examination Procedure with Patient in the Sitting Position 16

Chapter IV Terminology 16

Chapter V The Normal Sonoencephalogram (SEG) 17
A. Origin of SEG Reflections 17
B. Initial Echo (IE) and End Echo (EE) 17
Thickness of the Osseous Cranium 17
C. Midline Echo (ME) 18
D. Demonstrating the Third Ventricle 19
Third Ventricular Reflections 19
E. Lateral Ventricular Echoes and Determination of the Ventricular Index 21
Lateral Ventricular Index (LVI) 22
F. Lateral Echoes (Temporal Horn Echoes, Insula Echoes) . . 25
1. Brain Mantle Index (BMI) 26
2. Comparison of Capability of Measuring LVI and BMI in Various Age Groups 27

Chapter VI The Abnormal Sonoencephalogram 28
A. Midline Echo Shift 28
B. Recognition and Identification of the Midline Echo . . . 29
C. Demonstrating the Dilated Ventricular System 30
D. Calculation of the Pathological Lateral Ventricular Index . 30
E. Measurement of the Abnormal Third Ventricle 32
F. Determination of Abnormally Enlarged Lateral Ventricles by Exhibition and Measurement of the Outer Wall of the Temporal Horn—Brain Mantle Index (BMI) 34

Part Two: Special Sonoencephalography

Chapter VII Brain Trauma 36
A. Sonoencephalographic Examination of Children with Post-Traumatic Intracranial Hematomas and Hygromas . . . 36
Brain Concussion and Contusion 36
B. Intracranial Hematomas 37
1. Epidural Hematoma 37
Hematoma Echoes 38
2. Acute Subdural Hematoma 38
3. Chronic Subdural Hematoma 39
4. Subdural Hygroma (Pachymeningosis serosa) 39
5. Intracerebral Hematoma 40
Illustrative Cases 41

Chapter VIII Sonoencephalographic Examination of Childhood Hydrocephalus 45
A. Examination of 188 Children with Clinically Suspected Internal Hydrocephalus 46

Chapter IX Sonoencephalographic Examination in Intracranial Space-Occupying Lesions 48
A. Supratentorial Space-Occupying Lesions 51
B. Infratentorial Space-Occupying Lesions 52

Chapter X Congenital and Developmental Defects and Brain Damage in Early Childhood 54
A. Sonoencephalographic Findings 55
B. Prenatally Determined Brain Damage as Sometimes Exhibited in Phenylketonuria 58

Chapter XI Sonoencephalographic Examination in Various Convulsive Disorders 64

Chapter XII Reliability of the Sonoencephalogram in the Diagnosis of Childhood Hydrocephalus 66
A. Comparison of SEG Results with other Clinical Data . . 68

B. Comparison of SEG and PEG Measurements of the Third Ventricle 72
C. Comparison of Sonoencephalographic and Pneumoencephalographic Values of the Lateral Ventricle 73
1. Calculation of the SEG Lateral Ventricular Index (LVI) 74
2. Evaluation of PEGs 74
3. Comparison of PEG and SEG Lateral Ventricular Index 75
D. Comparison of the Roentgenological and Sonoencephalographical Lateral Ventricular Index 77
E. The Value of SEG Follow-up Studies in Evaluation of Hydrocephalus 78
Illustrative Cases 79

Chapter XIII Sources of Error and Particulars 83
A. Erroneous Measurement in Determining the Midline Echo . 85
B. Sources of Error in Measuring the Width of the Third Ventricle 85
C. Sources of Error in Determining the Lateral Ventricular and Brain Mantle Index 85

Part Three: The Combined EEG and SEG

Chapter XIV The Combined Electroencephalographic and Sonoencephalographic Examination 87
A. Introduction 87
B. Sonoencephalographic Examination Procedure 88
1. Position of Diencephalic Midline 88
2. Determination of Lateral Ventricular Expanse 88
3. Measuring Third Ventricular Width 89
C. Subject Material 89
D. EEG Results 90
E. SEG Results 91
F. Comparison of SEG and EEG Findings 92
Illustrative Cases 94

References 109

Subject Index 134

Introduction

Sonoencephalography has evolved into a highly refined examination method since 1955 when Leksell first published a feasible method of examining cerebral structures with ultrasound.

This relatively new examination method is especially appropriate for the diagnosis of childhood intracranial disorders, since the boney structures of the immature skull absorbs substantially less sound energy than those of the adult cranium. This provides the most favorable conditions for optimum utilization of this method. However, the very nature of the immature skull of the child can cause sonoencephalographic reflections that are easily misinterpreted and misdiagnosed.

In order to establish normal values for diagnostic purposes and to correctly interpret reflections constantly appearing on the oscilloscope screen, 400 children were systematically examined ranging in age from earliest infancy to 16 years. The acquired normal values for the lateral ventricles, third ventricle and the diencephalic midline were compared to those obtained by other authors.

In addition, we have described a method of evaluating the lateral ventricles which is applicable in any clinic, as well as in a practice.

Sonoencephalography has proven to be a valuable diagnostic aid in childhood hydrocephalus, intracranial space-occupying lesions, intracranial hemorrhage, convulsive disorders of every etiology, congenital CNS defects, cerebral damage during early childhood, and cerebral atrophy. Sonoencephalographic detection of cerebral atrophy sometimes accompanying untreated phenylketonuria is given special consideration.

An entire chapter is devoted to the value of combined electro- and sonoencephalographic examinations. The presence or absence of focal EEG abnormalities and midline echo shifts can be of valuable assistance in the differential diagnosis of intracranial disorders.

In conclusion, we would like to point out one of the main assets of the sonoencephalographic method; namely, that in many cases it completely eliminates employment of potentially dangerous methods utilizing contrast media. It is a convenient, accurate, and harmless method which can be performed either on an outpatient basis or within the clinic.

Part One: General Sonoencephalography

I. General Physical Properties of Sound in Liquids and Gases

Mechanical waves in elastic media are termed sound waves. In solids these appear as longitudinal and transverse waves. In liquids and gases only longitudinal waves can exist, since these media do not possess shear elasticity necessary for transverse oscillations. In longitudinal wave motion, displacement of particles of the medium results in compression and expansion of the medium, whereas in transverse waves their displacement results in deformations of the lattice of the medium.

Wave length λ is the shortest distance between two particles that are in the same phase or state of motion.

The number of cycles of motion (either longitudinal or transverse) a particle completes in one second is termed the frequency, f. The time necessary for one cycle of motion is the period T of the wave. Period and frequency are connected by the simple equation

$$T = \frac{1}{f} \text{ [sec]} \tag{1}$$

The unit of frequency f is sec^{-1}. 1 sec^{-1} is usually termed 1 cps (cycles per second).

The propagation velocity c of a wave is its phase velocity, i. e., the traveling velocity of a particular state of motion. Between propagation velocity, wave length and frequency we have the following relationship:

$$c = \lambda \cdot f \quad \text{(general wave formula)}$$

$$\begin{aligned} \text{where } c &= \text{propagation velocity [cm} \cdot \text{sec}^{-1}] \\ \lambda &= \text{wave length [cm]} \\ f &= \text{frequency [sec}^{-1}] \end{aligned} \tag{2}$$

Propagation velocity c depends upon the physical characteristics of the medium and on the temperature.

Sound velocity in gases is given by Laplace's equation

$$c = \sqrt{\frac{1}{\varrho \cdot \varkappa}} \tag{3}$$

Since $\varkappa = \frac{1}{\frac{c_p}{c_v} \cdot p}$, we obtain $c = \sqrt{\frac{c_p}{c_v} \cdot \frac{p}{\varrho}}$. $\varkappa$ is the modus of compressibility of the gas at constant temperature and c_p and c_v are the specific heats of the gas at constant pressure and volume, respectively. ϱ is the density and p the pressure. The value of c_p/c_v for air is 1.4. At O °C and p = 760 mm Hg (standard atmospheric pressure), the density ϱ of air is 0.001293 g/cm³. Thus, for air we obtain the sound velocity at 0 °C; $c_0 = 33{,}113$ cm/sec.

In gases, the velocity of sound depends upon the temperature in the following manner:

$$c_t = c_0 \sqrt{1+\alpha \cdot t} \qquad \text{where } c_0 = \text{velocity at } 0\,^\circ\text{C}, \; t = \text{temperature in } ^\circ\text{C}, \; \alpha = \text{constant } (=1/273.2\,^\circ\text{C}) \text{ for air} \qquad (4)$$

Sound velocity in liquids is calculated by

$$c = \sqrt{\frac{1}{\varrho \cdot K}} \qquad \text{where } \varrho = \text{density}, \; K = \text{modulus of adiabetic compressibility} \qquad (5)$$

In solids sound velocity is calculated by

$$c = \sqrt{\frac{E}{\varrho}} \qquad \text{where } E = \text{modulus of elasticity} \qquad (6)$$

A sound wave transports energy which is stored in the vibrational motion of the particles of the propagation medium. Sound intensity I is defined as the amount of energy incident on a surface area of 1 cm² in 1 sec,

$$I = \frac{E}{s \cdot t} \qquad \text{where } E = \text{energy in erg}, \; s = \text{surface area in cm}^2, \; t = \text{time in sec} \qquad (7)$$

In order to represent the extreme range of sound intensities and to correlate these with our perception of intensity, the term decibel is employed. The intensities I_1 and I_2 of two sounds differ by 1 decibel (db) when the decadic logarithm of their ratio, multiplied by 10, has the value 1. This means that I_1 exceeds I_2 by x db when

$$10 \log_{10} \frac{I_1}{I_2} = x$$

Consequently, in specifying an absolute sound intensity in decibels one always refers to a reference level.

Roughly, it can be said that the subjectively perceived sound volume V is proportional to the logarithm of the objective physical stimulus, i. e. the sound intensity (Fechner Weber Law),

$$V \propto \log I$$

In order to define V more exactly, one proceeds in the following manner: the strength of a sound (volume) is measured by comparing it to a reference tone of 1000 cps which is perceived at the same loudness. The objective intensity of that standard tone of 1000 cps, measured at the ear, is compared to the standard intensity of $I_0 = 10^{-16}$ erg/(cm² sec) of the standard tone which is just sufficient to evoke auditory perception (hearing threshold) i. e., the volume is defined as

$$V = 10 \log_{10} \frac{I}{I_0} \qquad (8)$$

V is a number without dimension and its unit is 1 phon.

Loudness	Phon
Whispering	10
Conversation	50
Pain	130

A. Classification of Sounds

According to human thresholds, physical sounds are categorized into various frequency ranges. Sound frequencies under 16 cps, which are inaudible to the human ear, are termed subsonic. Frequencies within the hearing range of 16 to approximately 20,000 cps are called audible sounds, and those above the hearing threshold, $>$ 20,000 cps, are termed ultrasonic.

B. Physical Characteristics of Ultrasound

As a source of ultrasonic waves, we shall describe the piezoelectric phenomena, since we are dealing with this type of sound generation in medical ultrasonic. With increasing frequency, sound takes on some of the physical properties of light, e. g., it propagates practically in a straight line. The piezoelectric sound source produces parallel sound beams over a short distance, termed the near-field, after which they begin to diverge. The initial plane wavefronts assume a spherical shape in the far-field. The apex of the far-field cone is the sound source. The length of the near-field L is proportional to the square of the radius (r) of the source and the frequency of the sound waves and inversely proportional to the velocity of sound propagation in the medium.

$$L = \frac{r^2 \cdot f}{c} \tag{10}$$

Enlargement of the near-field is accomplished either by increasing the sound frequency or by increasing the diameter of the sound source or both. From equation 10 it can be demonstrated that when a sound probe with a diameter of 15 mm and a frequency of 2 Mcps is employed, a near-field of 73.5 cm is obtained when a propagation velocity of 1.53×10^3 m/sec for brain tissue is accepted.

C. Laws of Reflection and Refraction

An acoustic interface is required for reflection, refraction, and dispersion of sound waves. Such an interface is characterized by two bordering media exhibiting different acoustical impedances. Acoustical impedance R (sound wave resistance) of a medium is defined as the product of the specific sound propagation velocity c and the characteristic density ϱ of that medium.

$$R = \varrho \cdot c \; [g \cdot cm^2 \, sec^{-1}]$$

The familiar laws of light optics (electromagnetic waves) can be applied to acoustical reflection, refraction and dispersion. Reflection is influenced by two dimensions: a) the angle of incidence at which the wave strikes the acoustical interface, and b) the acoustical impedance of the two media involved. When an ultrasonic wave strikes the acoustical interface at an angle, one portion of the wave (as well as one portion of the intensity) is reflected and the other portion is refracted. Since the optical law of reflection is valid, the angle of incidence α_1 is equal to the angle of reflection α_2. The index of refraction n can be obtained by Snell's law.

$$n = \frac{\sin \alpha}{\sin \beta} = \frac{c_1}{c_2} \tag{11}$$

According to the law of energy conservation, the intensity (I_0) of the incident sound wave is equal to the sum of the intensities of the reflected intensity (I') and the intensity (I'') entering medium 2.

$$I_0 = I' + I'' \tag{12}$$

According to the following equation, the reflected intensity is a function of the acoustical impedances R_1 and R_2 of the media 1 and 2 as well as of the angle of incidence α and of the angle of refraction β.

$$I' = I_0 \frac{R_2 - R_1 \frac{\cos\beta}{\cos\alpha}}{R_2 + R_1 \frac{\cos\beta}{\cos\alpha}} \tag{13}$$

Similarly, the intensity entering medium 2 is represented by

$$I'' = I_0 \frac{4\, R_1 \cdot R_2 \frac{\cos\beta}{\cos\alpha}}{\left(R_2 + R_1 \frac{\cos\beta}{\cos\alpha}\right)^2} \tag{14}$$

D. Conditions Favorable to Reflection

Since the sound probe serves as transmitter as well as receiver in sonoencephalography, only those sound waves can be registered on the oscilloscope screen that are reflected into the area of the probe. This holds true only when the ultrasound beam is projected perpendicularly to an interface, since, at relatively small deviations from the normal, reflected sound waves by-pass the probe.

In further consideration, we can view the angle of incidence as negligibly small and consider perpendicular propagation as well as perpendicular reflection from an interface to be valid.

When an ultrasonic beam strikes an interface perpendicularly, one portion will be reflected in the direction from which it originated, and the other portion will enter the second medium without being refracted. With $\alpha = \beta$ and hence $\frac{\cos\beta}{\cos\alpha} = 1$, we can conclude from equations 13 and 14 that:

$$I' = I_0 \left(\frac{R_2 - R_1}{R_2 + R_1}\right)^2 \tag{15}$$

and

$$I'' = I_0 \frac{4\, R_1 \cdot R_2}{(R_2 + R_1)^2} \tag{16}$$

According to equation 15 the reflected intensity increases as the difference in the acoustic impedance of the two media increases.

In cases where the two interfaces involved represent identical acoustical impedances, $R_1 = R_2$, then $I' = 0$, i. e., no sound will be reflected and the entire intensity is transmitted into the second medium ($I'' = I_0$). When differences in acoustical impedance are large, i. e., when R_2 is much larger than R_1 or, inversely, when R_1 is much larger than R_2, the ratio $\left(\frac{R_2 - R_1}{R_2 + R_1}\right)^2$ approaches the limit value of 1. In this case, the reflected intensity approaches the transmitted intensity ($I' \simeq I_0$) and practically no sound is transferred to medium 2.

Table 1. *Acoustical impedance of various substances and tissues*

Medium	Acoustical impedance [$g \cdot cm^{-2} \cdot sec^{-1}$]
Air	48.2
Water	$150 \cdot 10^3$
Glycerine	$240 \cdot 10^3$
Steel	$470 \cdot 10^4$
Muscle	$163 \cdot 10^3$
Fat	$136 \cdot 10^3$
Bone	$610 \cdot 10^3$
Dura	$172 \cdot 10^3$
Brain	$156 \cdot 10^3$
Liquor	$151 \cdot 10^3$
Blood	$166 \cdot 10^3$

It can be observed from Table 1 that air has the smallest acoustical impedance of all media reported. On an air-tissue interface almost complete reflection occurs. This observation is of special importance in ultrasonic diagnostics.

E. Diffraction

When the ultrasonic beam strikes an obstacle, say a small disc of diameter d, the marginal waves undergo diffraction. The angle of diffraction is given by

$$\sin\alpha = \frac{\lambda}{d} \qquad \text{where } \lambda = \text{wave length} \tag{17}$$

At the periphery of acoustical interfaces, similar refraction of marginal waves into the shadow zones occurs. The angle of diffraction is proportional to the wave length λ and inversely proportional to the dimensions of the obstacle.

When the wave length λ is small compared to the obstacle's dimensions, the angle of refraction is correspondingly small, and the refracted waves are nearly canceled by interference. Behind such a hindrance, the sound waves propagate straight, producing a distinct shadow.

When the wave length and the dimensions of an obstacle are in the same order of magnitude, the typical refraction patterns are obtained behind the obstacle.

F. Sound Scattering and Absorption (Sound Attenuation)

In inhomogeneous media the ultrasonic beam strikes many particles which possess larger or smaller acoustical impedances than their surroundings. Such particles represent many acoustical interfaces whose borders diffract marginal sound waves.

The angle of incidence of each wave comprising the ultrasonic beam is different when the beam strikes an interface surface of sufficient irregularity. Therefore, the angle of refraction and the angle of reflection of each wave are different, and the parallel sound beam is scattered.

Sound scattering is proportional to the frequency and to the density of irregularities of the interface. When the density of irregularities is large, sound scattering increases as the number of such surface irregularities increases, i. e., the ultrasonic beam is considerably attenuated.

An ultrasonic beam traveling through a (homogeneous or inhomogeneous) medium gradually decreases in intensity along the traveled path, since the energy stored in the vibrational motion of the particles is gradually transferred into heat. The sound wave undergoes absorption.

The decrease in intensity can be described by the following equation:

$$I_x = I_0 \cdot e^{-\beta x} \quad \text{where } I_x = \text{intensity at a distance x from the point at which the intensity is } I_0, \quad \beta = \text{coefficient of absorption} \tag{18}$$

This means that the intensity decreases in accordance with exponential function. The absorption coefficient increases with the frequency, i. e., the larger the frequency the shorter the distance at which the intensity has decreased, e. g., $I_0/2$.

II. Technical Considerations of the Ultrasonic Impulse Apparatus

Ultrasonic diagnostics presents a method by which internal tissue structures of the body can be represented on film. The type of films obtained from such an examination is determined by the technical construction of the ultrasonic echo apparatus. An ultrasound examination can produce an unidimensional picture (A-scope technique) or a two-dimensional picture (B-scope and C-scope techniques). The future is definitely more promising for two-dimensional sonoencephalography, since it has already been successfully employed in ophthalmology, internal medicine, surgery, and obstetrics and gynecology. Two-dimensional sonoencephalography poses several problems; namely, attachment of the probe, the individually variating thickness of the osseous cranium, and the complicated anatomical structure of the ventricular system. Valid results have been obtained only in children, since in such subjects the boney structures of the head are still quite thin. Because of these problems, the unidimensional method will continue to predominate in clinical sonoencephalography. We will consequently limit our discussion of the two-dimensional method and concentrate chiefly on the unidimensional examination (A-scope).

A. Construction of the A-scope Apparatus

The following simplified schema (Fig. 1) presents a general view of the construction and function of an impulse echo apparatus with the A-scope technique.

An impulse echo apparatus with the A-scan technique is composed of the following elements:

1. transmitter (high-frequency oscillator, sound probe),
2. receiver (sound probe, amplifier),
3. synchronization unit,
4. indicator gauge (cathode-ray tube),
5. sweep generator.

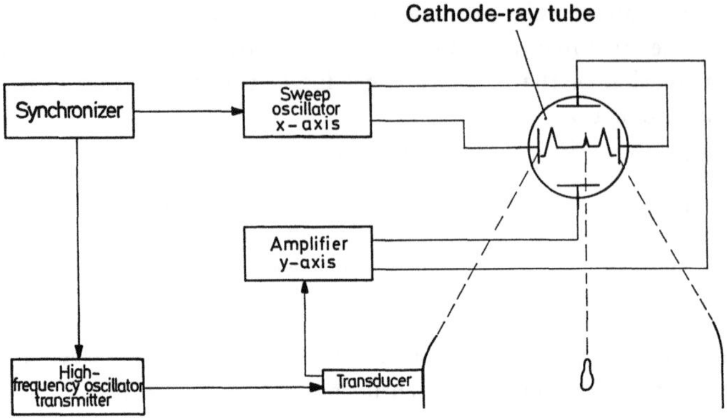

Fig. 1. Simplified block diagram with the most important circuit elements: synchronizer, high-frequency oscillator, transducer, amplifier, sweep oscillator, and cathode-ray tube. The cathode-ray tube demonstrates a sonogram from a sketched portion of the body

The above components must fulfill the following requirements in order to produce a valid picture of internal tissue structures:

1. Transmitter

The ultrasonic transmitter is composed of a high-frequency oscillator and a sound probe.

a) High-frequency Oscillator. The high-frequency oscillator serves to produce electrical impulses in the ultrasonic sound range. In sonoencephalography, frequencies between 1 and 2 Mcps have proven practical and sufficient. However, in ultrasonic diagnostics of soft tissue areas, as practiced in obstetrics and gynecology, relatively wider frequency ranges divided into 1, 2, 4, and 6 Mcps are employed. Because of the high degree of resolution, sound frequencies ranging between 6 and 15 Mcps are necessary in sono-ophthalmology.

b) Sound Probe (Transducer). The sound probe serves to transform high-frequency electrical impulses into mechanical impulses, i. e. ultrasonic pulses. The most important component of the sound probe is the piezoelectric crystal. By varying the voltage applied to two adjacent surfaces, the crystal is stimulated to perform volume vibrations. A ceramic oscillator composed of lead zirconium titanate is most widely employed as a piezoelectrical crystal. Such ceramic oscillators produce the best results to date in medical diagnostics, since they generate the shortest pulse and possess high sensitivity. The shortest possible pulses are necessary, since the duration of the sound pulse determines the resolving power. The resolving power is defined as the capability of distinguishing between two echoes transmitted in rapid succession, i. e., whether the receiver registers two rapidly transmitted echoes separately, or as one extended single echo. Dependence of the resolving power on the pulse duration will be briefly described on the basis of the following two assumptions:

a) that one pulse echo with a half-width of 2 μ sec reaches the receiver within a time interval of 2 μ sec, and

b) that two pulse echoes, each with a half-width of *1 μ* sec, reach the receiver within the identical time interval.

The two echo pulses with a half-width of 2 μ sec will not be registered separately at the receiver. It can be observed from this example that by reducing the pulse duration by a factor of 2, the resolving power increases by the same factor. This means that tissue structures can be examined in more detail.

The most practical pulse duration of mechanical vibration is 0.1 to 1 μ sec. In order to keep the pulse duration at a minimum, a damper unit is fixed to the reverse side of the piezoelectric crystal. The result obtained with this procedure is that the mechanical vibration decreases within the shortest possible time period, and only a wave of short sequence is emitted. In order to improve radiation properties, a $\lambda/4$ adapter film and an epoxy resin lens are attached to the front of the piezoelectric crystal. These components contribute to sound bundling and are principally responsible for the production of the near-field.

2. Sound Receiver

The receiving component is essentially composed of a sound probe and an amplifier.

a) Sound probe (transducer). The ultrasonic probe functions both as transmitter and receiver. Such a sound probe is technically termed a transducer. After emission of the transmission pulse, the sender is "dead". We observe the base line on the oscilloscope screen when no reflections occur. During this "dead time" the probe functions as a receiver. The returning sound pulse enters the probe as an echo of the transmitted impulse and is quickly transferred into mechanical vibrations by the piezoelectric crystal. Since the piezoelectric crystal is capable of reacting to mechanical deformations by producing surface charges, and vice versa, the capacitor which is connected to the surface of the piezoelectric crystal receives a charge pulse which is transmitted farther, amplified and registered. Hence, the transducer functioning as a receiver transforms mechanical oscillatory pulses into electrical oscillatory pulses. That the transducer can interchangeably function as transmitter and receiver is solely due to the reversible physical properties of the piezoelectric crystal; namely, to react to surface potential oscillations with mechanical vibrations and to mechanical vibrations with surface potential oscillations. The pulse transmitting frequency is adjusted so that during the time interval between two successively transmitted pulses, all the echoes of the first pulse can be registered.

b) Amplifier. Sound waves decrease in intensity when penetrating a medium. Several factors are responsible for this loss which can also be effective in sound distribution within the human body. These factors include the following: 1. increasing divergence of the wave beam with increasing distance from the sound source. Consequently, smaller energy distribution per surface unit occurs with increasing distance from the sound source. 2. Sound reflection from a strong reflecting interface inhibits deeper penetration of the sonic wave into the examination area. This is especially important in sonoencephalography, since the osseous cranium reflects with considerable intensity. Before penetration of the brain itself, the sound beam must consecutively transect the scalp, osseous cranium and the dura. 3. Dispersion from tissue inhomogenities, and 4. sound absorption, i. e., the loss of sound energy by heat production along the traveled path. The reduction in sound intensity through absorption is demonstrated in the following formula:

$$I_x = I_0 \cdot e^{-\beta x}$$

where I_0 represents the initial sound intensity (for $x = 0$), x the traveled path, I_x the sound intensity after traveling the distance Δx, and β the coefficient of absorption. e is the basis of the natural logarithm. The absorption coefficient β is dependent on the type of tissue and is proportional to the sound frequency. The latter means that a smaller amount of sound intensity is absorbed at lower frequencies than at higher frequencies and that the penetration depth is increased at lower frequencies.

When it is assumed that sound velocity and absorption are constant for the entire examination area, the sound intensity loss from absorption can be removed by *traveling-time-controlled amplification,* i. e., the amplification is controlled according to

$$A = A_0 \cdot e^{-\beta x}$$

where A_0 = amplification and x = penetrating depth in tissue, which is linked with the velocity c of the echo pulse and the traveling time t by $x = c \cdot t$. In this manner, echo amplitude that will be independent of tissue depth can be obtained.

However, it is a rare exception when sound velocity and absorption within an examination field are constant. Nevertheless, by velocity-controlled amplification it is possible to attain and register sound pulse echoes originating from even the most profound areas. This improves considerably the reliability of our results.

3—5. The Screen Image (Synchronization Unit, Indicator Gauge and Sweep Generator)

A cathode-ray oscilloscope is employed as an indicator apparatus. In order to produce a stable image on the oscilloscope screen, saw-tooth voltage is employed as x-sweep voltage which is provided by the sweep voltage generator. The saw-tooth voltage is synchronized with the pulse sequence. The increasing saw-tooth voltage causes the cathode beam to travel on the screen from left to right; the sudden decrease in the saw-tooth voltage causes the cathode beam to jump back from the right side to the left side, etc.

The screen image (i. e., the echogram or the sonogram) reproduces the time distances between the echoes and between an echo and the transmitted pulse. These time distances (Δt) are measurable and can be transformed into location distances (Δx) by the formula $\Delta x = c \cdot \Delta t$. The distances between locations or between echoes are identical to distances between locations of two or more sound interfaces within the examination field. A presumption for this interpretation is, of course, that the sound velocity remains constant along the traveled path. Naturally, this is not the case, since the existence of one echo already signifies that an interface is present which separates two different media with different sound propagation velocities. Therefore, the registered echo distances on the oscilloscope screen can only be qualitatively interpreted to represent the true distance of interface locations within the examining area. Quantitative evaluation cannot be determined, but can only be performed by exact knowledge of the various sound propagation velocities in the bordering media. This includes the assumption that, in subjects with simular sonograms, the velocity of sound propagation in the media between each echo is the same, or of such small variations that they can be considered irrelevant. With this assumption, comparative measurement can be performed, which is the topic of this book.

Since we performed the scanning procedure in each examined subject from the same direction and on the same part of the body, the above assumptions for two different sonograms can be related according to the following formula:

$$c_{12} = C'_{12} \quad \text{and} \quad c_{01} = c'_{01}$$

where c_{12} is the velocity of sound propagation in the medium of the body to be compared, which lies between the second spike (E_1) and the third spike (E_2). Similarly, c_{01} is the velocity of sound propagation between reflections E_0 and E_1 (Fig. 2).

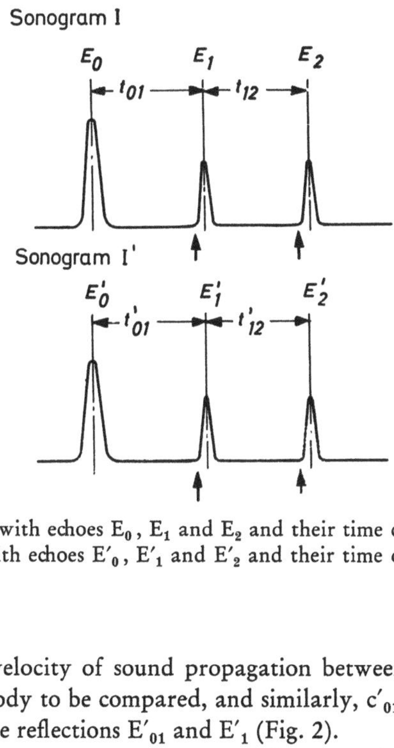

Fig. 2. Sonogram I with echoes E_0, E_1 and E_2 and their time distances t_{01} and t_{12}. Sonogram I' with echoes E'_0, E'_1 and E'_2 and their time distances t'_{01} t'_{12}

c'_{12} represents the velocity of sound propagation between reflections E'_1 and E'_2 in the medium of the body to be compared, and similarly, c'_{01} is the velocity of sound propagation between the reflections E'_{01} and E'_1 (Fig. 2).

With our assumption, we can now equate the ratios between the velocities of sound propagation in both bodies to be compared with the following formula:

$$\frac{c_{12}}{c_{01}} = \frac{c'_{12}}{c'_{01}} = \text{constant} = K$$

The time interval Δt_{01} and Δt_{12} between the echoes in the sonogram to be compared are related to the distances Δx in location in the compared bodies by the formula $\Delta x = c \cdot \Delta t$.

Therefore, $\Delta x_{12} = c_{12} \cdot \Delta t_{12}$

and $\Delta x_{01} = c_{01} \cdot \Delta t_{01}$

The same applies to the time distances $\Delta t'_{01}$ and Δt_{12} of the sonogram to be compared and the distances of locations in the comparative body:

$$\Delta x'_{12} = c'_{12} \cdot \Delta t'_{12}$$
$$\Delta x'_{01} = c'_{01} \cdot \Delta t'_{01}$$

When the ratios of echo distances from different sonograms are calculated, the following results:

$$\frac{\Delta x_{12}}{\Delta x_{01}} = \frac{c_{12}}{c_{01}} \cdot \frac{\Delta t_{12}}{\Delta t_{01}} = K \cdot \frac{\Delta t_{12}}{\Delta t_{01}}$$

accordingly,

$$\frac{\Delta x'_{12}}{\Delta x'_{01}} = \frac{c'_{12}}{c'_{01}} \cdot \frac{\Delta t'_{12}}{\Delta t'_{01}} = K \cdot \frac{\Delta t'_{12}}{\Delta t'_{01}}$$

It is now possible to directly relate variations in time ratio to variations in distance ratio: the latter are proportional to the former. When one accepts the conditions in healthy individuals as being standard conditions (experimental series), it is possible to detect the existence of abnormal conditions and the extent of such conditions by deviations from these standard conditions.

In the A-scope procedure, a unidimensional "picture" is obtained which is specifically predictive of tissue structures momentarily in the sound field. The probe can be moved in a definitive direction, and in this manner, a sequence of unidimensional pictures is obtained from which a two-dimensional or three-dimensional picture could be conceived with much effort.

In order to directly produce a two-dimensional picture, the amplitude modulation method (a-scope = amplitude scope) must be replaced by the brightness modulation method. Amplified echo impulses are not recorded on the y-deflection, but on the Wehnelt cylinder which regulates the intensity of the electron beam of the oscilloscope.

Two-dimensional ultrasound techniques are chiefly categorized into 4 methods:

1. linear-scan
2. arc-scan
3. sector-scan
4. compound-scan.

B. Linear-Scanning

In linear-scanning, the probe is moved in a straight line over the body component to be examined. The y-deflection on the cathode-ray oscilloscope is synchronously tuned to movement of the probe in a straight line. For each point along this path, a line with various brightness intensities is obtained on the oscilloscopes screen. The desired two-dimensional picture, represented by densely bordering lines, is obtained when all points along the path of the probe are scanned. Fluorescent film, which illuminates for a long period of time, is needed for the oscilloscope screen in order to stabilize the picture, since the time required for a picture assembly is the same as the time required for scanning the object (above 10 sec). This requirement applies as well to other two-dimensional ultrasonic techniques.

One difficulty in linear-scanning seems to be faulty coupling. A direct probe-skin connection is hardly possible, since the human body presents a rather uneven examination surface. Water is employed as a coupling medium between the probe and the body surface. While this type of coupling is associated with difficulties in practice, it has been successfully employed in ultrasonic ophthalmology.

C.—E. Arc-, Sector- and Compound-Scanning

Only an imperfect oscilloscope picture will result from linear-scanning, since only tissue interfaces positioned parallel to the course of the probe will reflect the ultrasonic pulses back to their source. However, not all tissue structures lie parallel to the course of the probe. It is consequently advisable to scan the tissue interfaces at different angles. In arc-scanning (Fig. 3, A), this is achieved by alternating the course of the probe into a circular arc.

In sector-scanning, the sound probe is held at a definite point permitting only sectorial displacement (Fig. 3, S).

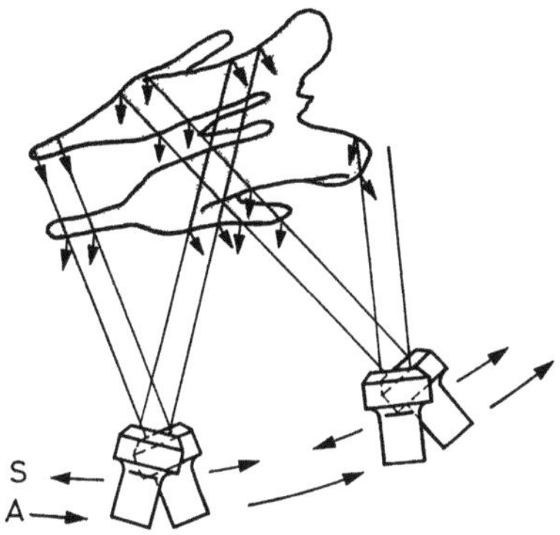

Fig. 3. Compound-scanning: the transducer is moved along a circular arc and is additionally swiveled around its own axis (perpendicular to the arc and to beam direction)

In compound-scanning (Fig. 3), arc- and sector-scanning are combined.

One shortcoming connected with linear-scanning, and to a lesser extent with arc- and sector-scanning, is that one point of an interface can be scanned from one direction only. Although this particular problem has been resolved by compound-scanning, other difficulties arise due to pulse dispersion.

Each point of an interface is struck from at least one direction. If a point reflects the pulse into the probe at some specific angle different from the angle at which the neighboring points reflect, the beam travels different distances. The traveling times of the echoes of a point and its neighboring points differ. Since the oscilloscope registers traveling times and not location distances, two neighboring points on an interface will be viewed displaced from one another. A distortion in traveling time occurs which impairs the image quality. However, there is no question that technical development of the two-dimensional ultrasonic technique is in its beginning stages.

III. Examination of Pediatric Patient

A. Examination Procedure with Patient in the Supine Position

The portable apparatus is first placed to the right of the patient's bed and switched on (Fig. 4). The time that it takes the impulse to appear on the oscilloscope screen gives the examiner the opportunity to disinfect his hands. Before the actual

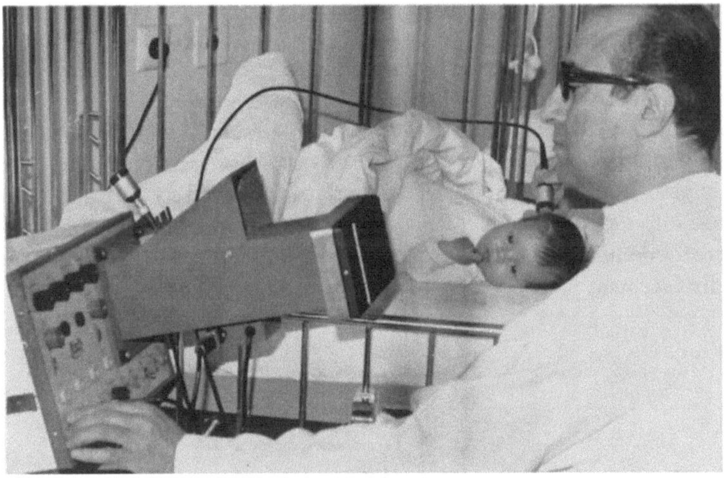

Fig. 4. Examination of a supine infant at bedside. (Kretz-Technik apparatus, series 4100 ME)

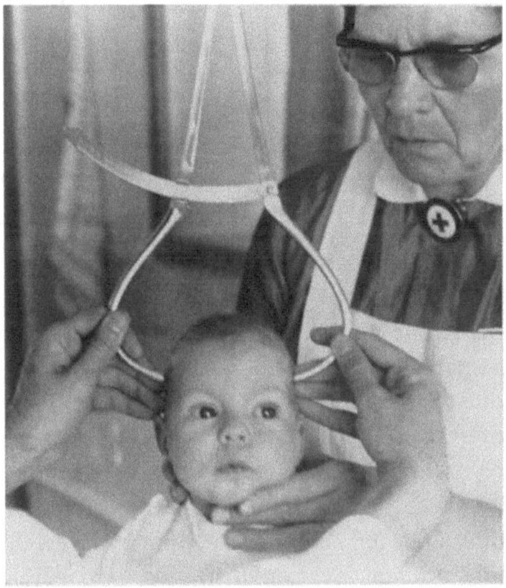

Fig. 5. Measuring the bitemporal cranial diameter of an infant in order to calculate the theoretical midline echo. Special observation should be given to the position of the fingers

examination begins, enough time should be taken in order to establish contact with the patient. In pediatrics this can be accomplished with a toy, which has the effect of calming the child and possibly alleviating his fears.

With the child lying on his back, the bitemporal diameter of the skull is measured with a set of callipers (pelvic calliper) (Fig. 5). Since the shape of the skull (especially in infants) is quite variable, it is always necessary to take at least two measurements from two different corresponding points of the squamous portion of the temporal bone.

The theoretical midline echo can be calculated from the arithmetical average of both measurements.

$$T = \frac{D_1 + D_2}{2} \qquad \text{where } T = \text{theoretical midline echo}, \quad D = \text{cranial diameter}$$

After suffusing the probe with a transmission substance, it is placed horizontally on the temporal bone slightly above the external auditory meatus. At this position, the ultrasonic waves are capable of transversing the cranium at a horizontal plane.

A quick orientation of the middle structures can easily be carried out from this examination position. From a distance of 2 to 4 cm above the ear, the septum pellucidum is registered on the oscilloscope screen from both sides of the skull. Next, a search is made for reflections from the outer walls of the third ventricle. In our experience with children, we have found that the third ventricle can be more easily recorded at a position directly above the ear, whereas it is usually found somewhat anterior to this position in the adult examination (Fig. 6).

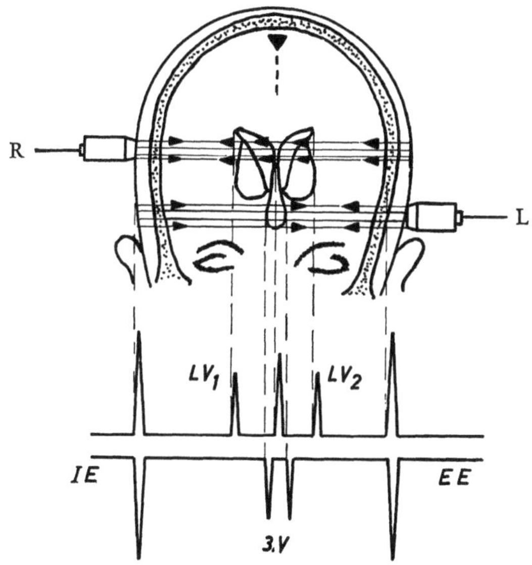

Fig. 6. Schematic representation of the origins of the echoes in a sonoventriculogram. Right (R): external reference point for demonstrating lateral ventricular echoes (LV_{1+2}). Left (L): external reference point and origin of third ventricular reflections

In order to view reflections from the walls of the lateral ventricles, the probe is positioned on the upper border of the temporal bone. It is very important that the head of the transducer be placed flush on the skin. By gently rocking the transducer against the scalp and viewing the oscilloscope screen, a search is then made for different components of the lateral ventricular complex.

In the examination of school children and adolescents, the same procedure is followed. If the patient remains calm, the examination can also be carried out with the examiner sitting at the head of the patient.

B. Examination Procedure with Patient in the Sitting Position

When the examination is performed on an outpatient basis, it is usually more convenient that it be carried out with the patient sitting or, in the case of infants and young children, with the patient sitting on the mother's lap. Older children can sit on a chair with a head rest. By positioning the head, the desired positions can be obtained so that the examiner may easily undertake the procedure from the right or left side of the head.

IV. Terminology

It is desirable that uniform nomenclature for Diagnostic Ultrasonics be established, and that the fixed terminology be internationally followed. We have accepted recommendations proposed by GROSSMAN concerning this terminology. GROSSMAN has suggested that all methods using the impulse echo procedure be termed *sonography*. Hence, the specific terms describing in detail the various ultrasonic procedures are all derivations of the word sonography, e. g., *sonoencephalography* (SEG) or *sonotomography*.

The term *A-scope* SEG is applied to unidimensional reconstruction of amplitude modulations recorded in the form of vertical deflections. The term *B-scope* SEG (brightness) is applied to unidimensional recordings in the form of dots.

All procedures using the unidimensional technique are expressed with the word "scope", whereas procedures using the two-dimensional techniques are termed "scan". The most important terms are A-scope and B-scan, since the unidimensional examination is normally recorded as amplitudes, and the two-dimensional as brightness intensity modulations.

The B-scope technique is employed mainly in cardiology; for example, in the examination of ventricular and valvular movements.

The *B-scan* technique is divided into the *linear B-scan* and *sector B-scan*, the difference being that the probe is moved in a linear direction during the former procedure and in the form of a sector from an immobile axis in the latter procedure (Fig. 3).

The term *compound-scanning* can be divided into *circular-* and *linear-arc-compound scanning*. In circular-compound-scanning the probe and the ultrasonic beam are moved radially around the patient. In linear-arc-compound scanning the probe is moved around the patient in a convex line without changing the direction of the beam.

A further differentiation can be made between contact-scanning and *water-path scanning*. In contact-scanning the probe is placed directly on the skin of the patient; in water-path scanning a water bath is positioned between the probe and the skin of the patient.

LEKSELL introduced the term *echoencephalography* for ultrasonic brain examinations. The abbreviation SEG for the sonoencephalogram has proven more practical for daily hospital practice than terms used by other authors. The term echoencephalography has found many contingents, but the abbreviation EEG is impractical, since it is identical with the abbreviation for electroencephalogram (EEG). The designation echo-EG is neither practical nor satisfactory.

We accept the terminological recommendations proposed by GROSSMAN, although complete conformity awaits the official decisions of an international congress.

V. The Normal Sonoencephalogram (SEG)

A. Origin of SEG Reflections

The standard reflections of the normal sonoencephalogram are produced when the ultrasonic beam-scalp angle is approximately 90°. The composite of reflections which appear to the far left on the oscilloscope screen is called the initial echo (initial complex, near-side echo, the "main-bang"). The reflection appearing in the middle of the field is termed the midline echo. The group of reflections at the far right is called the end echo (bottom echo, far-side echo).

B. Initial Echo (IE) and End Echo (EE)

The oscilloscope picture is typified on the left side by the initial echo (IE). In order to produce this complex of echoes, the ultrasonic beam must transverse several structures (hair, skin, bone, dura and the brain parenchyme itself). Consequently, a complex of reflections rather than a single spike appears as the initial echo. By varying the pulse intensity according to the age of the patient, the amplitude of the initial complex will be higher than the middle echo. The end echo, which has its origins from the inner table of opposite cranial wall, is also represented by a high-amplitude complex composed of 3—4 spikes (SMYTH).

Thickness of the Osseous Cranium

In the temporal procedure of sonoencephalography, the thickness of the boney structures of the head can be determined from the end echo complex. If the area of the scalp opposite the position of the transducer is massaged, egression of the reflections having their origins from these anatomical structures can be observed. By this procedure, it is possible to separate the portion of the end echo complex representing only the true end echo, which originates from the periost. This method of determining the true end echo was first proposed by DEVLIEGER.

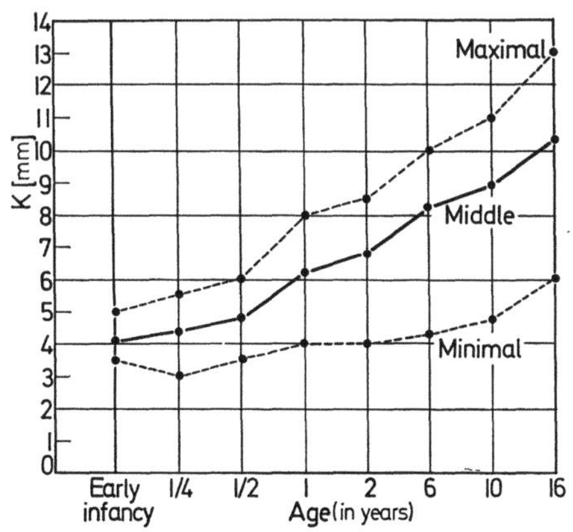

Fig. 7. Calculation of osseous cranium thickness (K) in various age groups

Measurement of the thickness of the osseous cranium is necessary in order to calculate the true cranial diameter (D), and to determine the theoretical midline echo. Such measurements have been performed by FEUERLEIN and DILLING, and SCHIEFER and KAZNER. Our results on measurement of the thickness of the osseous cranium in 400 children appear in Fig. 7. The solid dots represent the arithmetical average for each age group, and the points above and below express maximal and minimal values. The deviation from the average increases from 4 to 11 mm with increasing age.

C. Midline Echo (ME)

The midline echo originates at any interface between structures of varying acoustical impedance in the medial region and can, consequently, be modified by such structures. For example, the midline echo can be produced by single reflections from the falx cerebri, the septum pellucidum (Fig. 8), or by double reflections from the interhemispheric space. In the case of the latter, the midline echo complex often

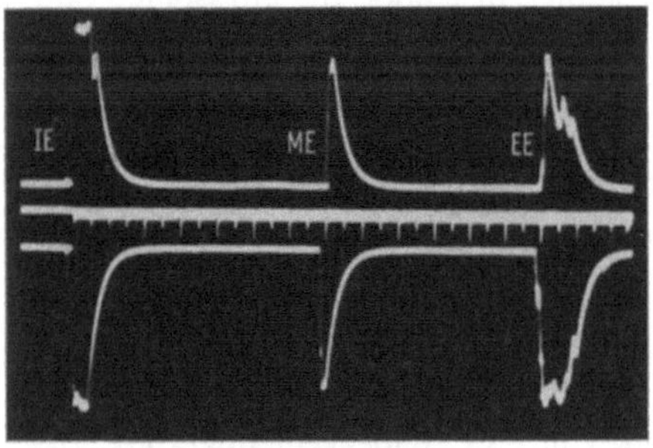

Fig. 8. Normal SEG film obtained from bitemporal scanning. IE = initial echo, M = midline echo, EE = end echo

exhibits a relatively wide base. The relationship of the measured midline echo to the theoretical (nominal) value enables detection of displaced medial tissue masses. The theoretical value for the position of the midline echo in each subject can be calculated from the SEG film in the following manner:

$$\text{Theoretical ME Value} = \frac{\text{expanse initial echo} \rightarrow \text{endecho} + \text{thickness of osseous cranium}}{2}$$

Midline shifts, such as those caused by hematomas, tumors, and subdural effusions, can easily be detected in this manner *(vide infra)*.

In our series of 400 healthy children, we were able to register the midline echo of each (Table 2). The midline echo was found to be absolutely in the middle in 347 of the children (86.75%). 51 subjects (12.75%) exhibited shifts up to 1 mm, and the remaining two patients (0.5%) showed shifts up to 2 mm.

The maximum midline shift considered to be within normal range varies from author to author. KAZNER and SCHIEFER view shifts of 1.5 mm in children as suspicious. They have recommended that further neuroradiological studies are indicated in such cases. On the other hand, JEPPSON (1961) considers a midline shift pathological when it exceeds 3.2 mm. Any displacement of the midline echo might be indicative of a space occupying lesion or unilateral cerebral atrophy although a displacement of 2 to 3 mm is frequently found in control cases.

Table 2

Age	Number of patients	ME bilaterally synchronous	ME shift up to 1 mm	ME shift up to 2 mm
Premature births and infants	110 (100%)	98 (89%)	10 (9.09%)	2 (1.8%)
Pre-school children	143 (100%)	121 (84.6%)	22 (5.4%)	— —
School-children	147 (100%)	128 (87.07%)	19 (12.9%)	— —
Total	400 (100%)	347 (86.75%)	51 (12.75%)	2 (0.5%)

The midline echo can pulsate synchronously with the heart beat in accordance with pressure variations in the cerebral fluid. The absence of such pulsations combined with decreased amplitude should be considered a prerequisite for the diagnosis of cerebral death (FISHGOLD et al.).

D. Demonstrating the Third Ventricle

The probe is placed on the lower part of the temporal bone without applying pressure. The position lies somewhat beneath the location from which the midline echo was demonstrated. By gently rocking the head of the transducer horizontally against the scalp, a group of three and occasionally four reflections can be found (compare ME). The medial reflection represents the ME, and the lateral spikes represent the corresponding lateral walls of the third ventricle (Fig. 9).

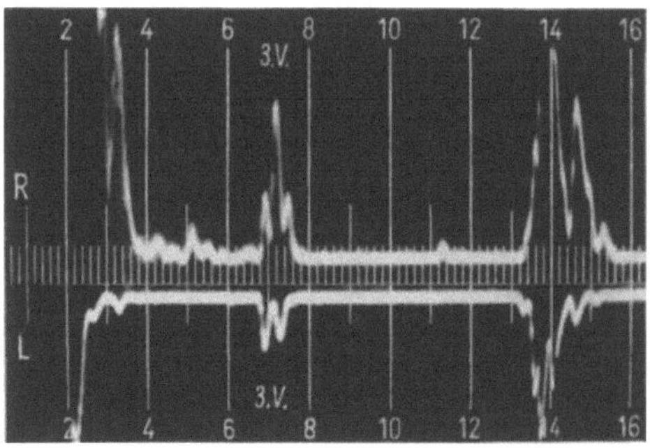

Fig. 9. The upper curve demonstrates three reflections originating from the third ventricle. The middle reflection represents the midline echo. A simple M-form echo signifies correct sonic beaming (lower curve). The distance between these two reflections represents third ventricular width (in the above case, 4 mm)

Third Ventricular Reflections

The different echoes comprising this complex originate from the interface of various structures of different acoustical impedance situated in the medial region and the grey and white matter, as well as from the cerebrospinal fluid-tissue interface. The question concerning the origin of these reflections has been studied by various authors (DEVLIEGER and RIDDER, 1959; TAYLOR, JEPPSON, BRAAK, W. G. TER, 1961; LITHANDER, 1961; SCHIEFER, KAZNER and BRÜCKNER, 1963; DREESE and NETSKY, 1964, etc.).

Deliverance of the ultrasonic beam from the correct external position and a favorable transducer-scalp angle enables the third ventricular complex to be registered on the oscilloscope screen in the form of a triple-pointed M or a simple M-form (Fig. 9). The distance between the two outer medial reflections denotes the width between the two lateral walls of the third ventricle and, consequently, can be considered a parameter for the size of the ventricle.

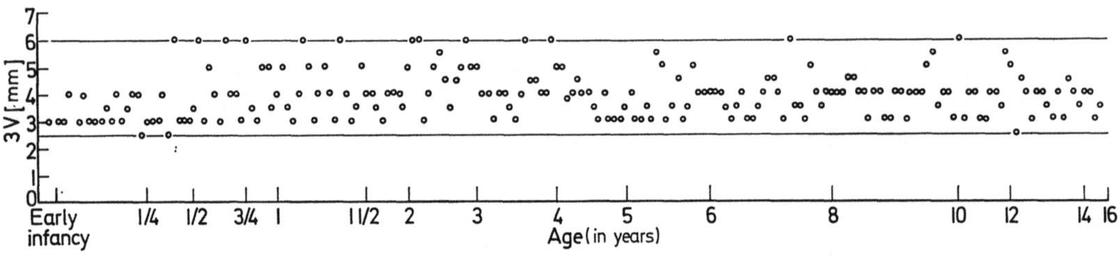

Fig. 10. Deviation range for third ventricular values of 200 normal children in various age groups

Observations on the anatomical shape of the third ventricle in vivo clearly demonstrate that the SEG values obtained depend on the portion of the ventricle from which the reflections originate. This fact must be considered when measuring the size of the ventricle, and when comparing the values obtained from different examinations and by different examiners. Due to the small size of the third ventricle in healthy children, correct SEG representation is difficult and frequently inaccurate.

The normal width of the third ventricle measured by other clinical methods, e. g., pneumoencephalography, has been studied by various authors. They differ considerably. For example, DAVIDOFF and DYKE consider 2.0 to 8.0 mm and ROBERTSON up to 9.0 mm to be normal. SEG measurements of the third ventricle have been carried out on healthy subjects of various ages by FEUERLEIN and DILLING. Their results lie within the range of 2.0 to 6.0 mm given by SCHIEFER, KAZNER, and BRÜCKNER. MOSTAFAWY et al. examined 400 healthy subjects from earliest infancy to adolescence. From this material 200 SEG films (50%), which fulfilled all criteria given in the literatur, were accepted. Figure 10 summarizes the findings for each age group. The lowest value was found to be 2.5 mm, whereas the majority exhibited values between 2.5 and 4 mm. Occasional values up to 6 mm were demonstrated. In our opinion, a diagnosis of third ventricular dilation should be made only when the 6 mm border has been exceeded.

Because of X-ray divergence, values for third ventricular width obtained in the pneumoencephalogram do not coincide with those obtained from the sonoencephalogram. By comparing 56 combined examinations, KAZNER and SCHIEFER (1966) were able to calculate PEG valus for third ventricular width up to 35% higher than those obtained from the SEG.

E. Lateral Ventricular Echoes and Determination of the Ventricular Index

In order to recognize reflections originating from the outer walls of the lateral ventricles, the ultrasonic beam must be placed so that it transcends the central part (cella media) of the lateral ventricles. This area can be found externally approximately 3 to 5 cm above the external auditory meatus on the superior border of the temporal bone. These reflections are visualized on the oscilloscope screen as a single spike on each side of the midline echo (Fig. 11).

The span between these lateral reflections and the midline echo is usually free from parenchyme echoes, since the ultrasonic waves transverse only the cerebrospinal fluid in this area.

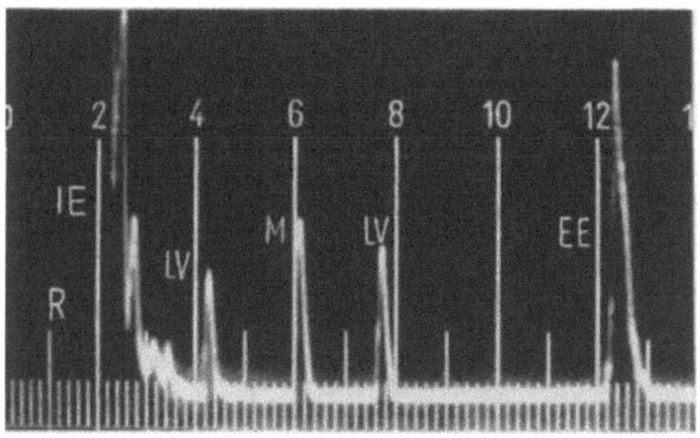

Fig. 11. Demonstrating the lateral ventricular reflections (LV) on each side of the midline echo (M). IE = initial echo, EE = end echo

Table 3. *Distance between the lateral ventricular reflections (d) as compared to the distance between the initial echo and end echo (IE → EE) in 320 children expressed in percentage*

Age distribution	Percentage	Total No.
Immature infants	27 to 31%	
1 to 6 months	22 to 33.6%, only in Case No. 364 35.9%	100 infants
7 to 12 months	22 to 31.8%	
1.1 to 2 years	23 to 32.0%, only in Case No. 376 34.1% Case No. 359 34%	115 young children
3 to 5 years	23.6 to 32.3%	
6 to 8 years	21.5 to 31.5%	
9 to 10 years	18.2 to 30.7%, only in Case No. 369 35%	
11 to 12 years	17.1 to 32.5%, only in Case No. 68 35.6%	105 school children
13 to 14 years	21.9 to 29.6%	
15 to 16 years	26%	

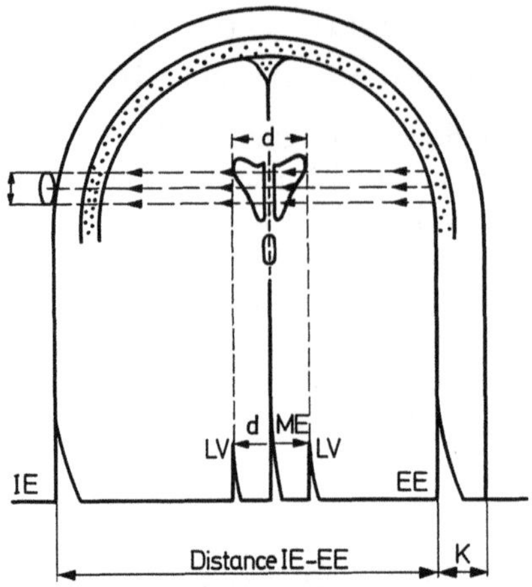

Fig. 12. Schematic demonstration of lateral ventricular index (LVI) calculation (modified after SCHIERSMANN): $\text{LVI} = \frac{\text{distance LV}_1 \text{ to LV}_2}{\text{distance IE to EE+K}} = \frac{d}{D}$
where D = cranial diameter, d = diameter of lateral ventricles, LV_1 and LV_2 = outer walls of the lateral ventricles, IE = initial echo, EE = end echo, M = midline echo, K = constant for osseous cranium thickness

The distance between the lateral ventricular reflections from the central body of each lateral ventricle varies; during childhood it represents about $^1/_3$ of the entire diameter of the skull.

From a series of 320 healthy subjects representing various age groups, we were able to measure the relationship between the reflections from the lateral ventricular walls and the span IE → EE. As is shown in Table 3, this relationship exceeded 35% in only 2 cases. SJÖGREN reported the distance between the lateral ventricular reflections of infants to be 33.5% ($^1/_3$ D) of the entire cranial diameter.

Lateral Ventricular Index (LVI)

Several authors have reported technical difficulties in obtaining true representation of the lateral ventricles and in the distribution of the width between the two lateral ventricles. Measurement of the temporal horn alone has been considered a more reliable parameter. On the other hand, other authorities such as J. SJÖGREN et al. have extensively described the ultrasonic representation of the lateral ventricles from the cella media. It has been recommended as particularly advantageous in follow-up studies.

It has been our experience that SEG measurement of the lateral ventricles of children has proven highly successful.

According to MOSTAFAWY et al. (1969), we utilized a ventricular index in our studies for evaluating the magnitude of the lateral ventricles. This index has been appropriatly termed the **lateral ventricular index (LVI).** Determination of lateral ventricular conditions by employing the sonoencephalographic LVI is undertaken in the following manner: from the SEG film, the distance between reflections originating from the outer walls of each lateral ventricle is measured (LV_1 to LV_2). This distance, which is termed d, is then expressed in relation to the corresponding cranial diameter, termed D. D is calculated by determining the distance from the initial echo complex to the end echo (IE to EE) and adding this to the thickness of the osseous cranium (as much as 10 mm) expressed as an age dependent constant K (Fig. 7). The dimension for d and D is millimeters.

As is expressed in Fig. 12, the lateral ventricular index is obtained by dividing the lateral ventricular width by the cranial diameter (modified Schiersmann index).

$$\text{LVI} = \frac{\text{Distance between the outer walls of the lateral ventricles}}{\text{Cranial diameter}} = \frac{d}{D}$$

d = distance between the two reflections representing the lateral ventricular walls

D = IE + EE + K

K = age dependent constant for the thickness of the osseous cranium

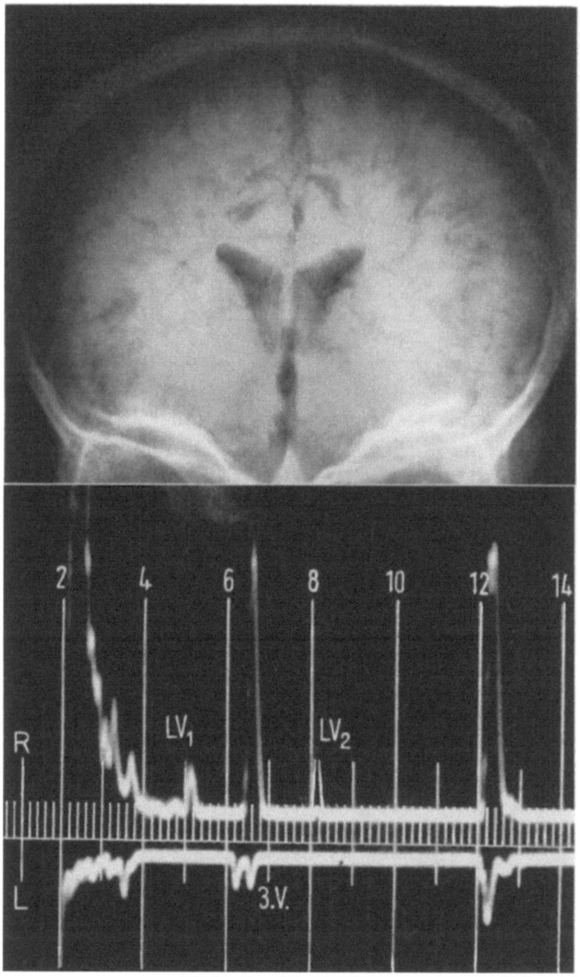

Fig. 13. Correlation in SEG and PEG findings in a 5 year old child with a normal ventricular system (lateral ventricular index = 0.24). LV_1 and LV_2 = lateral ventricles, 3. V. = third ventricle

An example follows:

Calculation of the lateral ventricular index from the sonoencephalogram of a one year old child (Fig. 13):

$$LVI = \frac{\text{Distance } LV_1 \text{ to } LV_2}{\text{Distance IE to EE+K}} = \frac{d}{D}$$

$$LVI = \frac{30}{121+5} = 0.24$$

Measurement of the lateral ventricles has also been undertaken by other authors such as WEST, SJÖGREN, UMBACH and KLEY, BRAHM et al., and LOMBROSO et al. SJÖGREN recommends the procedure only during the first year of life. Employing a method different from ours, BRAHM et al. determined the magnitude of the lateral ventricles in 115 children up to 16 years of age. However, their method has not found much support, since it is too complex for routine examinations.

We have examined the following group of 400 "healthy" children, varying in age from earliest infancy to 17 years, in order to measure lateral ventricular echoes (Table 4).

Table 4. *Age and number of patients examined in order to measure lateral ventricular echoes*

	Age	Number
Infants	up to 12 months	110
Pre-school children	1 to 5 years	143
School-children	6 to 16 years	147

Children with known or suspected neurological or mental defects were not accepted in this series. We were able to determine the distance between the outer walls of the lateral ventricles without difficulty in 320 of 400 subjects (80%).

The upper curve (LVI) of Fig. 14 represents the percentage of patients in whom we were able to measure the echoes from the outer walls of the lateral ventricles, and consequently, calculate the lateral ventricular index. Fig. 14 demonstrates that the lateral ventricles of premature infants are the most favorable to examination (100%). In early childhood the possibility was reduced to 70%, and at the age of 14 only about 60% of the measurements could be carried out.

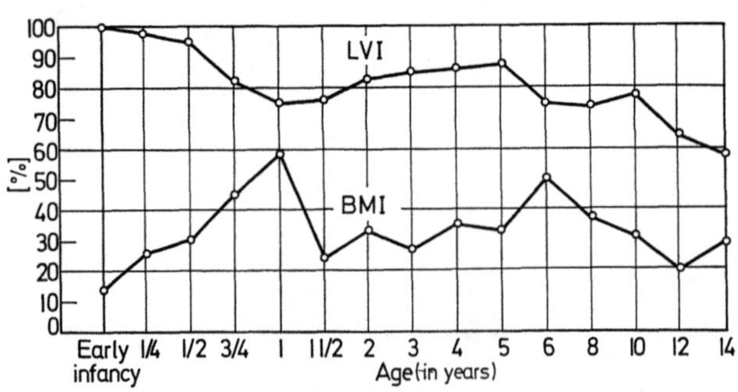

Fig. 14. Percentage distribution of the capability of measuring the lateral ventricular index (LVI) and brain mantle index (BMI) in various age groups

It must be stressed that the time required for a flawless SEG examination of the lateral ventricles of healthy children increases proportionally with the age of the patient.

The values for lateral ventricular indices calculated from these measurements are given in Fig. 15. Normal values, ranging from 0.20 to 0.32, were determined in a series of examinations comparing sonoencephalographic and air encephalographic measurements.

In this series four children were found to have values above the border of 0.32, and an additional four exhibited values below 0.20. Our limit of 0.32 for the upper norm corresponds to the value of 0.33 measured by J. Sjögren when taking into account differences in procedures.

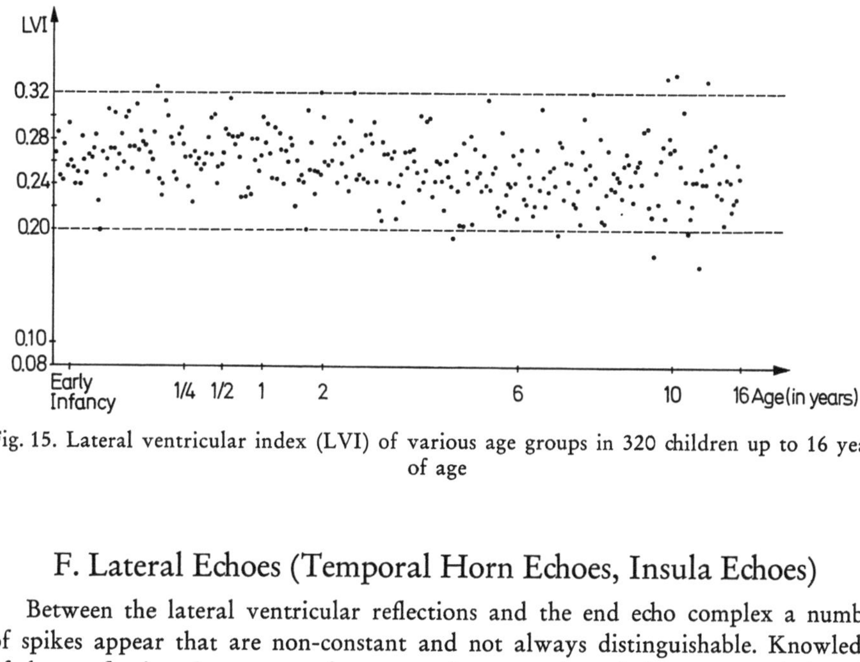

Fig. 15. Lateral ventricular index (LVI) of various age groups in 320 children up to 16 years of age

F. Lateral Echoes (Temporal Horn Echoes, Insula Echoes)

Between the lateral ventricular reflections and the end echo complex a number of spikes appear that are non-constant and not always distinguishable. Knowledge of these reflections is necessary for correct interpretation of the sonoencephalogram. Lateral reflections not only have their origin from the temporal horn (inferior horn) of the lateral ventricles, but also — occasionally — from one of the following structures:

1. temporal lobe (from the so-called insula cisterna)
2. nucleus lentiformis
3. internal capsule.

The temporal horn echoes are clinically the most important and will be dealt with in more detail. These are represented by two low-parallel spikes which originate from the inner and outer table of the temporal horns. In the bitemporal examination they appear on the oscilloscope screen when the probe is positioned so that the ultrasonic beam is directed slightly to the back of the skull in a downward position (Fig. 16, beam direction).

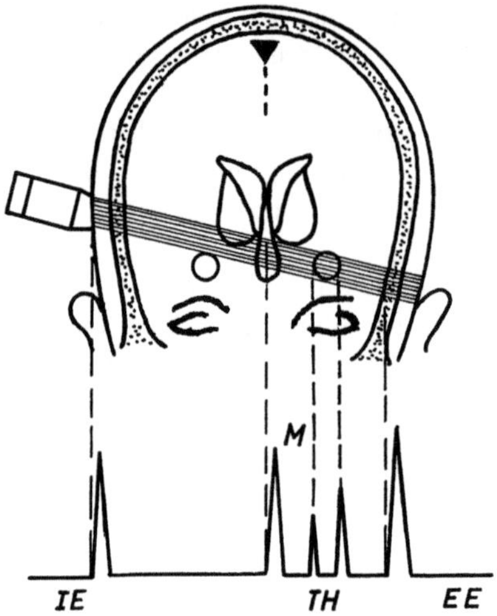

Fig. 16. Examination procedure in demonstrating temporal horn (TH) echoes

1. Brain Mantle Index (BMI)

By employing the temporal horn echo from the hemisphere opposite the probe, SCHIEFER, KAZNER, and KUNZE (1965) established the brain mantle index (Fig. 17). In order to calculate the BMI, the following two measurements from the SEG film are placed in relationship:

a) the distance from the midline echo to the end echo (a), and

b) the distance from the echo originating from the outer wall of the temporal horn to the end echo (b).

In other words, BMI $= \frac{a}{b}$.

The authors reported 2.0 to 2.2 to be the normal range of values. Findings above 2.4 were considered pathological.

Recognition and clear representation of the echoes from the lateral wall of the temporal horn is difficult when the ventricular system is not dilated. Moreover, additional reflections in children from this region (insula cisterna, etc.) further complicate the situation. Correct interpretation of these findings depends to a large extent on the experience and practice of the examiner. SCHIEFER and KAZNER compared pneumoencephalographic measurements of the temporal horn to those made by the SEG. They obtained confirmation of SEG results in 110 of 114 patients (97%).

M. JACOBI calculated the BMI of 108 healthy children and reported the following results: 92 subjects exhibited values between 2.0 and 2.2, 10 were reported to be 1.9, and 6 patients were found to have values between 2.3 and 2.4. The range of normal values was considered to be 2.0 to 2.2, with 2.3 being considered the upper borderline.

From our series of 400 children exhibiting no clinical manifestation of CNS disease, we were able to measure the reflections from the lateral walls of the temporal

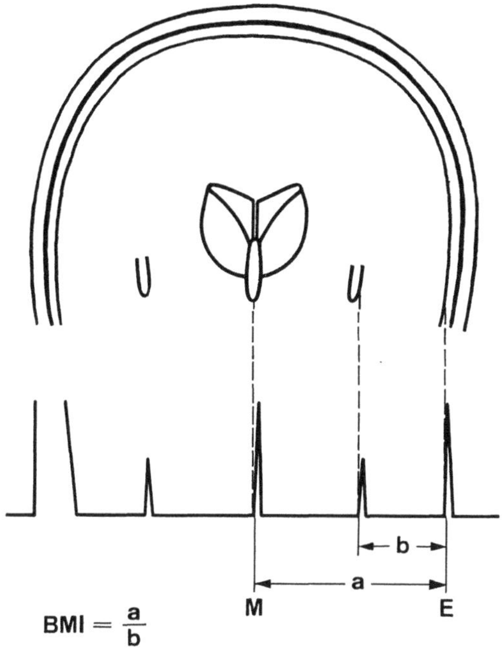

Fig. 17. Diagramatic representation of SEG brain mantle index (BMI) calculation. (From KAZNER, SCHIEFER and KUNZE, 1965)

horn in only 128 children. SCHIEFER and KAZNER consider 2.4 to be the upper border for brain mantle indices. We were able to confirm the border value of 2.4. With the exception of one patient with a value of 2.5, all results were within this range. The possibility of registering the reflections necessary for measuring the brain mantle index in different age groups varies. KAZNER was able to determine the BMI in 90% of the cases with ventricular enlargement. In our series of children with normal ventricles, the BMI was measurable in only 32% of the subjects.

2. Comparison of Capability of Measuring LVI and BMI in Various Age Groups

The lower curve of Fig. 14 represents the percentage of patients in whom definite representation of the reflections from the lateral wall of the inferior horn was possible (BMI). Comparison of this curve with the upper curve representing the capability of measuring lateral ventricular indices (in earliest infancy 100%) demonstrates that the capability of measuring the BMI in the same age group is usually 30% lower. During early childhood, measurement of the BMI increases to about 50% at six-years of age and the LVI decreases to 70% for the same age group. The capability of measuring either BMI or LVI decreases with increasing age up to 14 years.

Comparison of the two curves indicates that the possibility of measuring the LVI in children is larger in each age group than the possibility of measuring the brain mantle index.

VI. The Abnormal Sonoencephalogram

A. Midline Echo Shift

Each increase or reduction in volume of a cerebral hemisphere gives rise to a midline shift in the corresponding or opposite direction.

A midline shift is produced by lateral displacement of the medially located septum pellucidum, third ventricle, or falx cerebri. Such shifts can also be demonstrated by pneumoencephalography and angiography (internal cerebral vein) (Figs. 47 b and 49 b). The magnitude of tissue displacement depends on several factors:

1. location of lesion,
2. morphology of lesion,
3. degree of associated cerebral edema,
4. time factor (rapidity of volume increase),
5. the atrophical process.

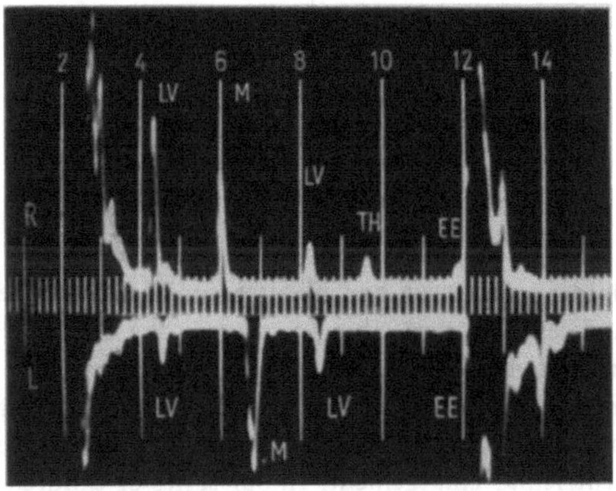

Fig. 18. Midline echo shift (MS) is represented by one-half of the difference between both midline echo measurements; where M right = b, M left = a. Therefore a+b = IE to EE. Midline echo shift in the above case is calculated as follows: MS $= \frac{66-60}{2} = 3$ mm to the right

An intracranial space-occupying lesion can be indirectly demonstrated by midline displacement. Direct documentation is possible when ultrasonic waves are reflected perpendicularly from the lesion interface. Consequently, it is possible to demonstrate various intracranial hematomas, cysts, intracerebral calcifications, and many types of neoplasmas, such as oligodendrogliomas and glioblastomas. These neoplastic tissue masses tend to undergo necrosis, calcification, and hemorrhage.

Distinct displacement of the supratentorial structures is expected only when the lesion is situated in the superior cranial fossa, since the solid connection between tentorium cerebelli and cerebral falx prevents massive displacement in the occipital area.

In order to calculate the magnitude of a midline shift (MS), the midline echo is measured from the right (a) and left temple (b). The "true" shift is half of the difference between the two measurements (a − b).

$$MS = \frac{a-b}{2} \qquad a+b = \text{IE to EE} \quad \text{(see Fig. 18)}$$

JEPPSEN (1961) and SCHIEFER and KAZNER (1967) consider shifts up to 2 mm as being normal values. LITHANDER (1961), PLANIOL et al. (1964), and KRAMER (1967) do not view midline displacements of 3 – 4 mm as being always significant. NICHOLS et al. (1968) consider shifts over 3 mm as significant. In our series of 400 healthy subjects varying in age from infancy to 17 years, we were unable to demonstrate shifts of more than 2 mm. Repetitious SEG midline shifts of over 2 mm must be viewed with suspicion. A complete survey of all SEG parameters is essential in establishing the diagnosis of massive tissue displacement, e. g.,

a) determination of third ventricular width, and

b) determination of the SEG lateral ventricular index.

B. Recognition and Identification of the Midline Echo

Any experienced examiner is capable of identifying the midline complex of healthy children (compare p. 18). The abnormal case presents even the most experienced examiner with diagnostic difficulties. When massive displacement is present, it is necessary to use additional criteria. Normally, the SEG midline appears as a single or double high amplitude reflection on the oscilloscope screen. LEKSELL (1955) wrote the following concerning the identification of this complex: "course and wide based pulse-synchronating amplitude pulsation." Although the midline echo of many children pulsates, it is our experience that this criteria is not a reliable aid to identification.

Accurate recognition of the midline echo depends upon anatomical knowledge of brain structures giving rise to the midline complex.

JEPPSON (1960—1961) considers the following structures responsible for the midline reflection: lateral walls of the third ventricle, posterior portion of the septum, and, partially, the interhemispheric space and the cerebral falx. Studies relating the origin of the midline echo to the pineal body have been performed by DEVLIEGER, RIDDER (1959), LITHANDER, and KARVOUNIS et al. (1961). Application of this theory in children must be regarded as improbable, since the pineal body is not yet calcified.

GROSSMAN (1966) and SCHIEFER et al. (1967) have pointed out several sources of error when complications arise in determination of the SEG midline:

1. incomplete connection or deficient contact between transducer and scalp,
2. the oscilloscope requires calibration,
3. incorrect positioning of the transducer,
4. low-amplitude echoes due to irregularities of the temporal bone. Increasing the intensity of the sonic impulse can possibly compensate for this.
5. Increased density of the osseous cranium (especially in older children). Changing to a probe of 1 to 2 Mcps usually compensates for this.

The following abnormal complications can give rise to difficulties in determining the midline complex in patients with an intracranial lesion:

1. presence of a "midline" tumor (located in the third ventricle, quadrageminal bodies or the basal ganglia),

2. presence of a space-occupying lesion in the temporal lobe,

3. hydrocephalus internus. This case can present a multitude of unidentifiable reflections. In extreme hydrocephalus the midline echo can be absent or of low-amplitude quality.

4. Congenital CNS defects and cerebral atrophy. The midline echo can be represented by several reflections.

When difficulties in identification of the true midline echo arise, it is advisable to calculate the theoretical midline echo (see p. 18).

C. Demonstrating the Dilated Ventricular System

The overall width of the cerebral ventricles increases proportionately with the age of the child. A reliable value for the upper limit of normal values has to date not been definitely defined. The different results of various authors can be attributed to several factors, including examination procedure and the reference line from which the examination was performed. Figs. 10 and 15 demonstrate that the uppermost borderline for normal values remains fairly constant, regardless of the age of the patient. It is not feasible to diagnose an enlarged ventricular system from results of the measurements of the third ventricle or the lateral ventricles alone.

When the SEG examination reveals values of 0.31 for the LVI and/or 6 mm for the third ventricle, it is advisable to then emphasize other clinical parameters such as cranial circumference, etc. Measurement of the lateral ventricular index from the cella media portion of the lateral ventricles was part of our preliminary SEG examination of each patient. The BMI was measured when reflections from the temporal horn could be demonstrated as a single entity on the oscilloscope screen.

D. Calculation of the Pathological Lateral Ventricular Index

Thin boney structures during childhood, which allow profound penetration of the ultrasonic waves, render the SEG ventricular examination relatively easy. By horizontally beaming the cella media from the superior border of the temporal bone, three characteristic and easily recognizable spikes appear (Fig. 11).

The magnitude of actual ventricular dilatation can be calculated by employing the SEG lateral ventricular index, which is a modification of the roentgenological index of Schiersmann. Fig. 12 demonstrates schematically the calculations necessary for determining the lateral ventricular index (LVI) as measured from the cella media. The following classification for LVI values over 0.30 has proven useful:

A) LVI up to 0.30 = normal lateral ventricles

B) Border range I: LVI between 0.30 and 0.31 = "bulky" lateral ventricles
   Border range II: LVI between 0.31 and 0.32 = "bulky" to slightly dilated lateral ventricles

C) LVI over 0.32 = definitely abnormal lateral ventricles

The following SEG of a 10 year old boy is an example (Fig. 19):

$$LVI = \frac{LV_1 \rightarrow LV_2}{IE \rightarrow EE + K} = \frac{57}{130+8} = 0.41$$ where K = thickness of osseous cranium

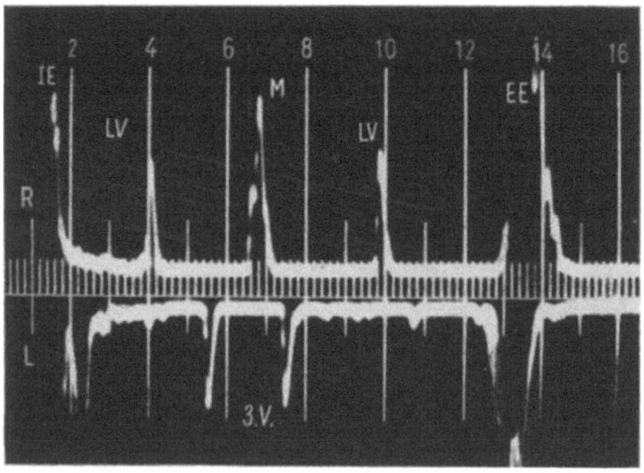

Fig. 19. Sonoencephalogram of a 10 year old with a distinctly enlarged ventricular system. Calculated values are as follows: lateral ventricular index = 0.41 and third ventricle = 18 mm

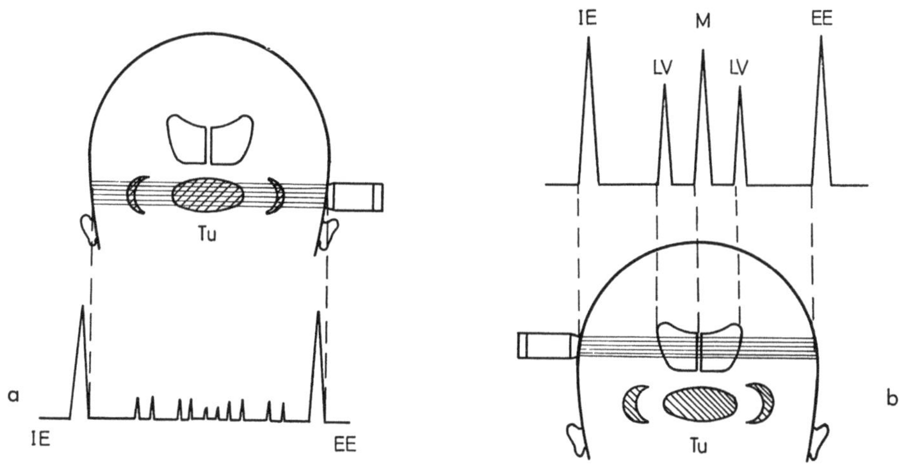

Fig. 20. Measurement of the third ventricle is complicated by additional reflections (tumor complex) when a tumor (Tu) in the thalmic area is present (a). In such cases, determination of the lateral ventricular index (i. e., lateral ventricular expansion) remains possible (b)

The lateral ventricles were definitely dilated in this case.

Measurement of the lateral ventricles can also be performed when determination of the third ventricle is complicated by an intracranial lesion in the thalmic area. Such a case is represented in Fig. 20. Increased reflections (e. g. tumor complex) can render identification of other SEG parameters impossible.

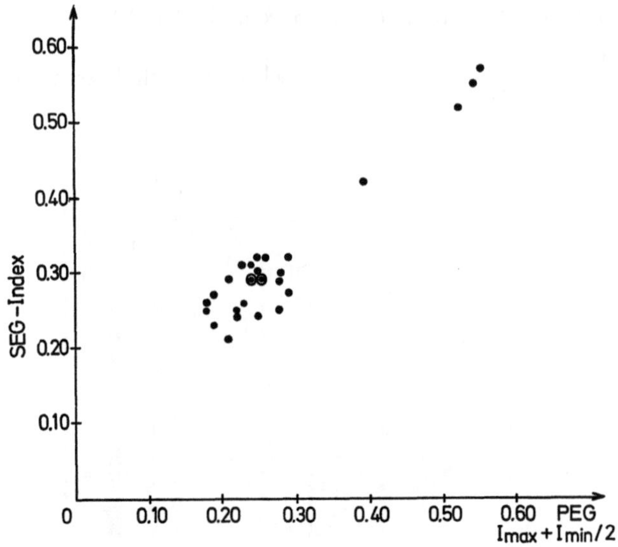

Fig. 21. Graphic representation of sonoencephalographic and pneumoencephalographic index values for the lateral ventricles with good correlation: SEG-Index $\frac{I_{max}+I_{min}}{2}$ = "r" = 0.95

Contrast examinations of the SEG and pneumoencephalogram (Fig. 21) demonstrate good correlation for LVI values ("r" = 0.95) (see Chapter XII). Since determination of the LVI can easily be carried out, it is also useful for the routine examination.

E. Measurement of the Abnormal Third Ventricle

Demonstration of reflections originating from the ventricular walls is especially practical during childhood, since the relative thin osseous cranium in children enables the sonic waves to pass easily.

By horizontally beaming the third ventricle from the external reference plane (see p. 19), a complex of 3 to 4 reflections appears in the midline area. With some practice and the correct transducer-scalp angle, these reflections are presented on the oscilloscope screen as a double echo (an "M"-shaped echo) (Fig. 9 and 22).

Pulsation of this complex is frequent during childhood, although not a requirement for identification.

The measurement can be read directly from the oscilloscope screen or, for documentation purposes, from the polaroid picture (Fig. 22). Each graduation mark on the base line scale in the picture represents 2 mm of brain tissue.

The distance between the two middle reflections denotes the width of the third ventricle, which increases with the age of the child. The uppermost borderline for normal values in infants up to 6 months has been given by Schiefer and Kazner as 4.5 mm. Initial studies performed by these authors on a group of 40 infants up to one year of age showed the highest value, exhibited by 6 patients, to be 5 mm. Further analysis of older children yielded values from 5.5 to 6 mm, which must be

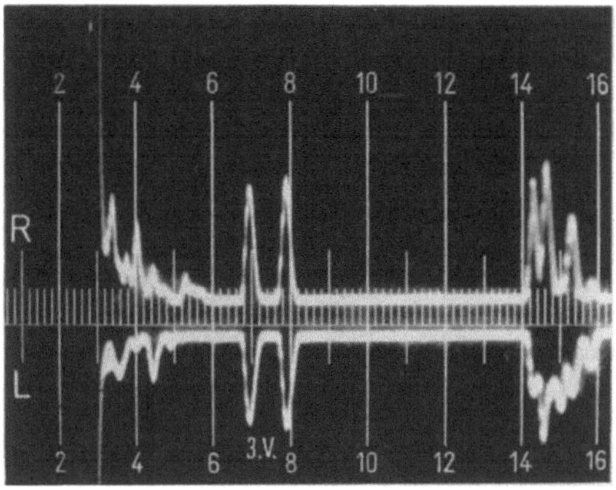

Fig. 22. Determination of abnormal third ventricular dilation in the bitemporal examination procedure. The distance between the two reflections represents third ventricular width. Each graduation on the baseline scale represents 2 mm of brain tissue. In the above case, third ventricular width is 9 to 9.5 mm

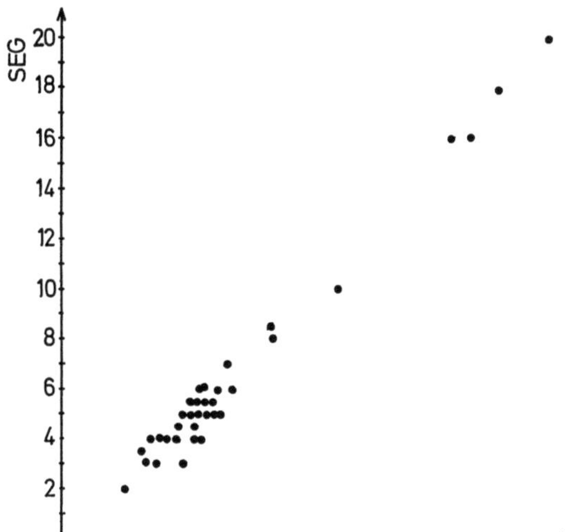

Fig. 23. Graphical representation of sonoencephalographic and pneumoencephalographic values for third ventricular width. A correlation of 94.6% is obtained when differences of ± 1.5 mm are considered; coefficient of correlation "r" = 0.93 and linear regression $y = 0.01105 + 0.90291 \cdot x$

considered still within the normal range. In normative studies by E. Jacobi, Schuch and Feuerlein and Dilling, almost identical results were reported.

We have measured the third ventricle in 200 healthy children varying in age from earliest infancy to 16 years (Fig. 10). Uppermost values of 6 mm were exhibited in 13 subjects ranging in age up to $10^1/_2$ years. We have thus used 6 mm as the uppermost borderline in this group. Since we obtained the value of 6 mm in 2 subjects from the group of school-aged children, the upper border of normalcy in this group was also determined to be 6 mm.

Comparison of combined SEG-PEG studies of the third ventricle has been performed by such authors as G. Jacobi, D. Schuch, Betz and Huber, Krüger, Zumpe, Veltin, Fliege and Backmund, and W. Feuerlein. In our combined SEG-PEG examination series of 37 cases, a correlation of ± 1 mm was exhibited in 83.8% of the cases (Fig. 23). When deviations of ± 1.5 mm are considered, 94.6% of the subjects are included. Two further cases demonstrated deviations of ± 2 mm in the two procedures.

Projection divergence in the X-rays, reported by Schiefer and Kazner to be from 25—35%, must be considered when comparing values obtained in the two procedures. This was accomplished by placing the PEG value for the third ventricle in relation to the PEG cranial diameter and multiplying this by the SEG cranial diameter.

A comparison of our results and those reported by other authors is presented in Table 5.

Table 5. *Comparison of correlation between combined PEG-SEG studies for the width of the third ventricle as reported by various authors*

SEG-PEG Deviation	Betz et al. %	Feuerstein et al. %	Jacobi et al. %	Krüger et al. %	Mostafawy et al. %
± 1 mm	59.2	73.3	68	75	83.4
± 1.5 mm	—	—	—	—	94.6
± 2 mm	82.4	96		96	100
± 3 mm	91.2	100		93	
± 4 mm					

Deviation in values obtained in the two procedures has been explained by Feuerlein and other authors by the following factors:

a) inconsistant external reference points,
b) the special anatomical form and position of the third ventricle, and
c) inaccurate measurement due to the apparatus.

F. Determination of Abnormally Enlarged Lateral Ventricles by Exhibition and Measurement of the Outer Wall of the Temporal Horn — Brain Mantle Index (BMI)

When ventricular dilation during childhood is suspected, a further SEG parameter is available to the examiner; namely, determination of the expanse of the lateral ventricular temporal horn. In order to perform this examination, reflections originating from the outer wall of the temporal horn are presented on the SEG film. Schiefer, Kazner, and Kunze were able to calculate the SEG brain mantle index (BMI) in the following manner:

$$\text{BMI} = \frac{\text{expanse midline echo} \rightarrow \text{end echo}}{\text{expanse temporal horn echo} \rightarrow \text{end echo}} = \frac{a}{b} \qquad \text{(Fig. 17)}$$

The external reference plane for this procedure is identical to that used in determination of the third ventricle (see p. 19). However, the sonic beam should not transverse the skull in a horizontal plane. The probe is slanted slightly downward in order that the sonic beam transects the walls of the probe-opposite temporal horn in a slightly cranio-caudal direction (Fig. 16). The echo from the outer wall of the temporal horn should appear on the oscilloscope screen half-way between the midline echo and the end echo. SCHIEFER et al. reported normal BMI values to be between 2.0 and 2.2, with abnormal values starting at 2.4.

The following is an example (Fig. 24):

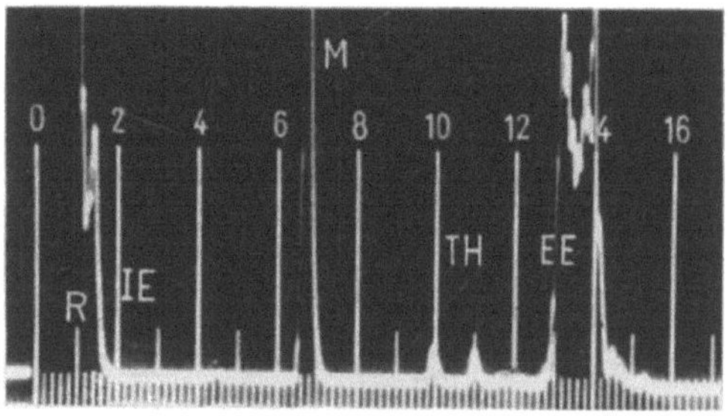

Fig. 24. Calculation of the brain mantle index (BMI) by demonstrating the outer wall of the temporal horn (TH).

$$\mathrm{BMI} = \frac{\text{distance midline echo to end echo}}{\text{distance TH to end echo}}$$

$$\mathrm{BMI} = \frac{65-129}{109-129} = 3.2$$

It has been mentioned that the midline echo in infants and pre-school children — especially in the abnormal cases — often appears as a double reflection that probably originates from the two outer walls of the third ventricle. In order to calculate the BMI in such cases, the mean distance between the two third ventricular echoes must be considered the position of the midline echo. Exactly such a case is presented in Fig. 42. The BMI calculation from Fig. 42 is as follows:

$$\mathrm{BMI} = \frac{67-130}{108-130} = 2.8$$

Correlation values of 97% for the BMI have been reported by SCHIEFER et al. in combined SEG-PEG studies. Therefore, the reliability of this determination can be considered significant. The procedure seems to be especially appropriate in the routine examination.

Part Two: Special Sonoencephalography

VII. Brain Trauma

A. Sonoencephalographic Examination of Children with Post-Traumatic Intracranial Hematomas and Hygromas

The sizable increase in street traffic in the recent past has been accompanied by a surge in the number of head injuries reported from traffic accidents. For example, in West Germany 150,000 to 200,000 body injuries are sustained yearly in traffic accidents. From this number approximately 50,000 can be considered serious head injuries; about 10,000 of these are associated with hematoma. In the United States, over 100,000 deaths each year may be directly attributed to head injury. More than 2.5 million such injuries necessitate some form of medical attention. Complications arising from head injuries, e. g., epidural and subdural hematomas with increased intracranial pressure on the affected side, demand immediate recognition. The sonoencephalogram has proven to be a valuable aid in the diagnosis of such lesions.

Brain Concussion and Contusion

Most all types of head injuries can present the same clinical picture as a *brain concussion*. Due to accompanying edema, post-traumatic M-echo shifts that seldom reach abnormal proportions ($>$2 mm) can be detected within a few hours in children. Tissue displacement associated with cerebral edema increases in the beginning and regresses completely after about two weeks. Discrepancy in position of the two end echoes obtained in the bitemporal examination must be detected in order to avoid misinterpretation of the position of the midline echo, which can occur post-traumatically as a result of a cephalic hematoma. In the presence of a subgaleal hematoma it is possible that the midline echo can be only unilaterally demonstrated.

In *brain contusion* midline echo shifts can be detected earlier and reach greater dimensions (on the average between 3—5 mm) than in concussion. Schiefer and Kazner reported one case with shifts up to 8 mm.

Post-traumatic transit dilation of the ventricular system can be detected by determination of the lateral ventricular index and measurement of the width of the third ventricle. These parameters should be constantly checked in SEG control studies until neurological symptoms subside and normal values are exhibited in the SEG.

We have examined 70 patients, varying in age from a few days to 16 years, with brain concussion or contusion (Table 6). On the second day after the trauma, we were able to detect massive tissue displacement of more than 2 mm in 4 cases (5.7%). In 5 subjects (7.2%), we were unable to measure the ventricular system.

In one of the above cases, the patient had undergone a birth trauma with hemorrhage into the spinal fluid. We performed a SEG serial study over a 4-week period after lumbal punctures, thereby observing a decline in the dilated lateral ventricles by determination of the lateral ventricular index (LVI = 0.52, LVI = 0.38). For a more detailed description of this case see Figs. 41 a and 41 b.

Table 6. *SEG results of 70 examinations performed on patients with a brain contusion or concussion*

Suspected diagnosis	No. of cases	Midline echo shift			Lateral ventricular index (LVI)			Third ventricle			Brain mantle index (BMI)			Hematoma echo		
Brain concussion or contusion		under 2 mm	over 2 mm	not measured	normal	over 0.30	not measured	normal	over 7 mm	not measured	normal	over 2.3	not measured	isolated	Echo-complex	not demonstrated
Grand total	70	65	4	1	61	4	5	64	1	5	26	5	39	1	—	69
Percent	100	92.8	5.7	1.5	87.1	5.7	7.2	91.3	1.5	7.2	37.1	7.2	55.7	1.5	—	98.5

B. Intracranial Hematoma

Intracranial hematomas can become manifest as an early or late complication of brain trauma. Close surveillance of such cases is absolutely necessary because of the danger of secondary hematomas and brain compression. By directly demonstrating *hematoma echoes* and detecting the presence of *tissue displacement*, the sonoencephalographic examination is capable of rendering great assistance in establishing a diagnosis in these cases.

LITHANDER (1961) attributed no diagnostic value to the SEG demonstration of hematoma echoes, especially in children. In more recent years, FORD and AMBROSE (1963); GELETNEKY (1964, 1965, 1966); BARROWS et al. (1965); and JACOBI, KAZNER and WOLLENSAK (1966) published results demonstrating the value of the SEG in such cases. GELETNEKY stressed the importance of bilateral hematoma echoes in the pediatric examination. SCHIEFER and KAZNER were able to demonstrate mild to moderate tissue displacement in 7 of 45 children with unilateral effusions.

1. Epidural Hematoma

An epidural hematoma is usually a sequelae of traumatic damage to the middle meningeal artery which results in bleeding into the epidural space. The blood cannot escape and, in turn, accumulates in a localized manner quickly producing increased pressure on the brain. Since the dura is practically fused with the normal cranial vault during infancy, epidural hematomas are infrequent until the second year of life. The pressure produced by a spontaneous collection of arterial blood is seldom sufficient to penetrate into the epidural space, except in cases where the osseous cranium is extremely thin. When the patient is in deep coma associated with definite brain damage, it is often difficult to laterally localize a hematoma in the clinical situation. Unilateral dilated pupils and a fracture line can only suggest lateral localization of the underlying lesion. Definite and exact localization of such a lesion is important in attempting to evaluate the prognosis of such patients. Consequently, in recent years sonoencephalographic examination, which can be quickly performed in any clinic, has become an important aid to the clinician.

Hematoma Echoes

In the bitemporal examination procedure, epidural hematomas exhibit an additional needlelike, isolated reflection which has been termed the *hematoma echo* by DeVlieger, Pia, Geletneky, etc. This echo is distinguished from that produced by a subdural hematoma in its relatively *high amplitude*. The echo represents the exact border brain, dura and blood.

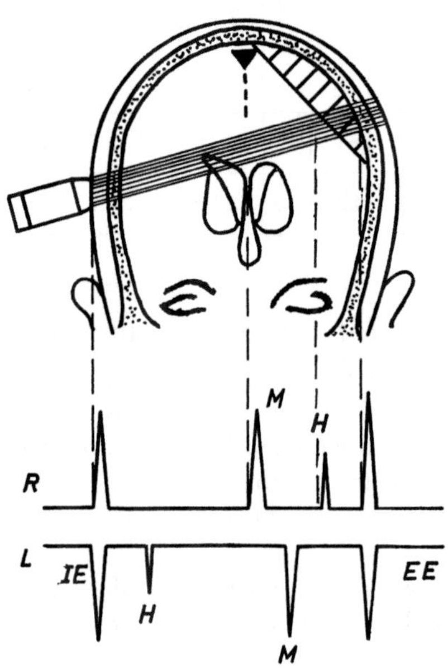

Fig. 25. Schematic representation of a hematoma echo and examination procedure in the case of an epidural hematoma in the parieto-temporal area. The spike (H) represents the border blood, dura and brain

In order to demonstrate a hematoma echo it is often necessary to rock the head of the transducer on the temporal bone until clear representation of the hematoma reflections from the probe-opposite side are recognized on the oscilloscope screen. The distance from the hematoma echo to the end echo represents the thickness of the hematoma. An epidural hematoma in the parieto-temporal area can often be demonstrated by slanting the probe (caudio-cranial examination, Fig. 25).

2. Acute Subdural Hematoma

Acute subdural hematomas usually become manifest as a brain contusion immediately after serious head injury resulting in hemorrhage. An exact clinical differential diagnosis between an acute subdural and an epidural hematoma is usually very difficult. Hemorrhage into the spinal fluid is always present in the former, although this finding does not rule out a simple contusion or a contusion accompanied by an epidural hematoma.

Brain damage associated with deterioration in the state of consciousness or unusually long periods of unconsciousness should always give rise to suspicion of an intracranial space-occupying hemorrhage. In order to correctly diagnose such cases, two methods of examination, both of which are harmless and easily performed, are available to the clinician; namely, the EEG and the SEG. Combined EEG-SEG examination quickly enables orientation on electrical activity of the brain and on the spacial relationship of the cerebral structures. Accordingly, it is possible to correctly diagnose many atypical hemorrhages and various intracranial space-occupying lesions with unusual clinical courses or neurological symptoms. In any case, lateral localization of the lesion can at least be determined (see Chapter XIV). Such information can be useful if carotid angiography is later performed.

In acute subdural hematoma the sonoencephalographic findings resemble those of an epidural hematoma, i. e., *tissue displacement*, on the average from 6 to 7 mm, and a *hematoma echo*. Contrary to the hematoma echo produced by epidural hemorrhage, acute bleeding into the subdural space produces an echo of *low amplitude*, since the well-defined reflections originating from the portion of the dura between the brain matter and hematoma are absent. In such cases the "dura echo" cannot be differentiated from the end echo complex in the usual manner. Identification of this particularity has little importance, since midline echo shifts have much more diagnostic value.

3. Chronic Subdural Hematoma

Clinically post-traumatic subdural hematomas are difficult to distinguish from hemorrhagic internal pachymeningitis, a term which is applied to the form associated with a pseudomembrane. Chronic subdural hematoma follows a traumatic incident in at least $^3/_4$ of all cases. The usual pathogenesis is tearing of the cerebral veins at their termination into the sagittal sinus. During infancy, subdural hemorrhage is usually the result of birth-related trauma.

In the SEG, displacement of the midline echo occurs in a manner similar to that found in association with epidural hemorrhage when the chronic subdural hemorrhage is unilateral. Occasionally a hematoma echo of low amplitude can be demonstrated.

Symptoms of chronic subdural hematoma may not appear for weeks or even months following even slight cerebral injury, whereas maximal manifestations are usually reached after 2 to 3 months. Older patients are usually involved. The clinical picture is dominated by headache; alternating levels of consciousness, with or without neurological symptoms; and xanthochromic liquor.

4. Subdural Hygroma (Pachymeningosis serosa)

Subdural hygroma is clinically almost impossible to distinguish from its predecessor, hemorrhagic internal pachymeningitis (Fanconi, Wallgren). It is usually composed of a thin collection of fluid over both hemispheres. A subdural hygroma can occur without trauma, and occasionally accompanies increased cerebro-spinal fluid pressure. It is bilateral in 85% of all cases, and occurs more frequently in infants between 2 and 4 months.

Sonoencephalographic examination reveals only slight displacement of tissue masses. In order to demonstrate the high-amplitude spiked reflections originating from such effusions, the probe must be placed so that the sonic beam is directed parieto-temporally (see Fig. 25). The usual position of this echo on the SEG film is directly before the end echo (Fig. 26), consequently, the distance between this echo and the end echo complex represents the degree of effusion. Aside from an effusion echo, considerable diagnostic value is placed on simultaneous measurement of the ventricular system. Dilation of the ventricular system has often been described in such cases; however, such dilation does not reach the proportions of childhood hydrocephalus.

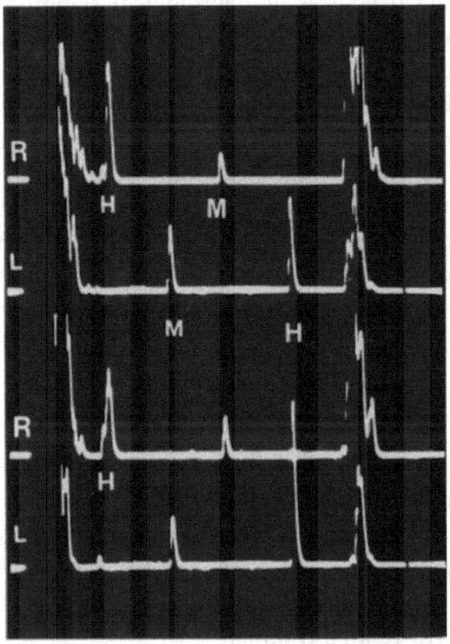

Fig. 26. The sonoencephalogram demonstrates a high-amplitude sharp-pointed effusion echo before the end echo in the parieto-temporal examination. The distance between this reflection and the end echo represents the expanse of the effusion (From SCHIEFER, W., 1967)

5. Intracerebral Hematoma

Intracerebral hemorrhage, which can occur by either rhexis or diapedesis type bleeding, usually produces a sudden and acute clinical picture. Clinical manifestations include abrupt increase in intracranial pressure accompanied by unconsciousness, increased motor tonus with cramping of the extensors, neurological signs of an intracranial lesion and, occasionally, fundoscopic abnormalities and tendency to asphyxia (K. A. BUSHE, P. CLEES).

Hemorrhage into the ventricular system (hematocephalus) is accompanied by a particularly serious prognosis, since rapid collapse of the vegetative regulatory functions quickly ensues in such cases.

An intracerebral hematoma is characterized in the SEG by the following findings:

a) midline echo shift representing diencephalic tissue displacement,
b) isolated hematoma echo, and/or
c) hematoma echo complex (Figs. 27 a and 25).

The degree of SEG-measured midline echo shift depends upon the location of the lesion in the brain. Schiefer and Kazner demonstrated an average M-echo shift of 5.5 mm in 14 subjects with unilateral intracerebral hematomas in the frontal lobe. When the location was reported to be in the temporal lobe, an average shift of 7.2 mm could be demonstrated in the SEG. Average shifts of 2.5 mm were reported when bilateral hemorrhage had occured.

Table 7. *SEG findings in 44 cases of acutely suspected intracranial hemorrhage*

Suspected diagnosis	No. of cases	Midline echo shift			Lateral ventricular index (LVI)			Third ventricle			Brain mantle index (BMI)			Hematoma echo		
Intracranial hemorrhage, subdural or intracerebral hematoma		under 2 mm	over 2 mm	not measured	normal	over 0.30	not measured	normal	over 7 mm	not measured	normal	over 2.3	not measured	isolated	complex	not demon-strated
Grand total	44	43	1	0	30	12	2	32	10	2	15	5	24	4	3	37
Percent	100	97.8	2.2	0	68.1	27.3	4.6	72.7	23.7	4.6	34.1	11.4	54.5	9.1	6.8	84.1

In our series of 44 children exhibiting signs of one of the various types of intracranial hemorrhages, we were able to demonstrate abnormal midline displacement in only one patient (Table 7). SEG values for the width of the lateral ventricles were found to be at the uppermost border or abnormal in 12 cases (27.3%). In 4 cases (9.1%), an isolated hematoma echo was demonstrated before the end echo; in one of these patients, bilateral hematoma echoes were discovered. In three further cases we were unable to determine abnormal midline displacement, although a hematoma echo complex was directly demonstrated (Fig. 27 a).

The following case histories should illustrate the value of the SEG examination in intracerebral hemorrhage.

Illustrative Cases

Case No. 1

Claudia S., $2^8/_{12}$ years old, admitted on Feb. 25, 1970, because of increasing dizziness and vomiting.

Case History: An influenza-like syndrome was reported 11 days before admission but was presumably without complications. Six days later blue spots began appearing over the entire body with increased petechial hemorrhaging. Increased dizziness and vomiting prompted clinical admittance in another city. During this admission extensor cramping, meningismus, and hemorrhage into the cerebrospinal fluid were reported. At this point the patient was transferred to our clinic.

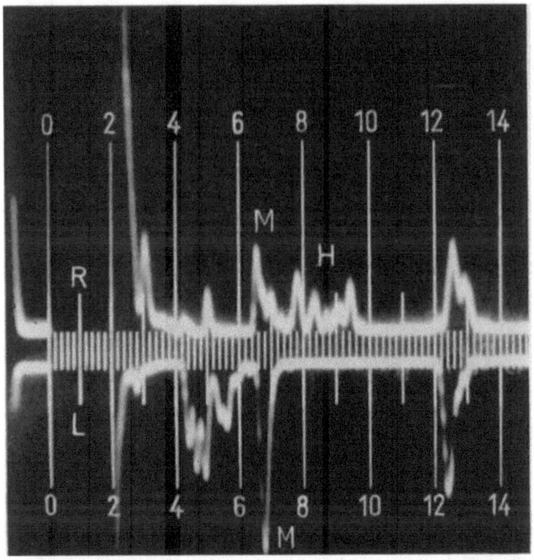

Fig. 27 a. Sonoencephalogram of a 2½ year old child with an intracerebral hematoma on the left side. Hemorrhage location is characterized by a group of additional reflections, the socalled hematoma complex (H), on the left side. Patient Claudia S., SEG No. 1550/70

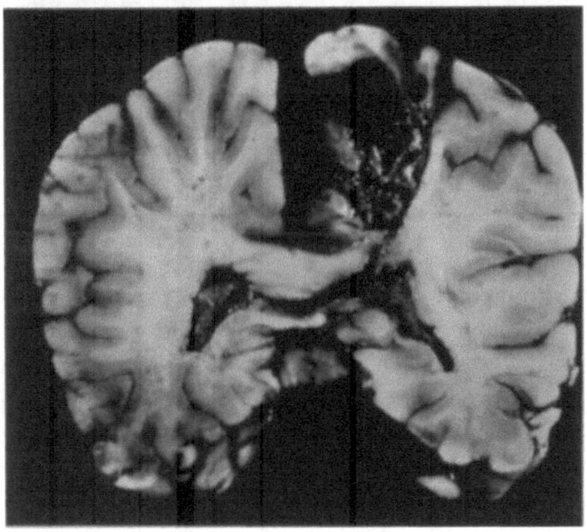

Fig. 27 b. Brain section from the same patient demonstrating the left sided hemorrhage. (Courtesy of Prof. G. Ule and Dr. K. Wagener, Institute of Pathology, University of Heidelberg)

Physical Examination: Unconscious child with constricted pupils on the right side and dilatated pupils unresponsive to light on the left side. Decreased muscle tonus, as well as deep tendon reflexes. Pyramidal signs were entirely absent. Petechial and massive hemorrhage over the entire body with principal locations on the tibia, knee, thorax, arm and head.

Laboratory Data: Hemoglobin 10.5%, erythrocytes 3.1 mil., leucocytes 16,700, thrombocytes 37,000. Increased coagulation time in the thromboelastogram and decreased prothrombin.

EEG: Base line EEG.

Fig. 28 A. Electroencephalographic follow-up study of a 5 month old infant (Case No. 2) with intracranial hemorrhage: a) Normal SEG before hemorrhage with basal activity corresponding to age (date, July 1, 1968). b) Distinct focus in the form of deceleration and depression over the left hemisphere during hemorrhage (date, July 27, 1968). c) Extensive normalization and disappearance of the focus after therapy (date, October 22, 1968). EEG of a 6 month old alert infant with intracerebral hemorrhage in constitutional thrombopathy

July 1, 68

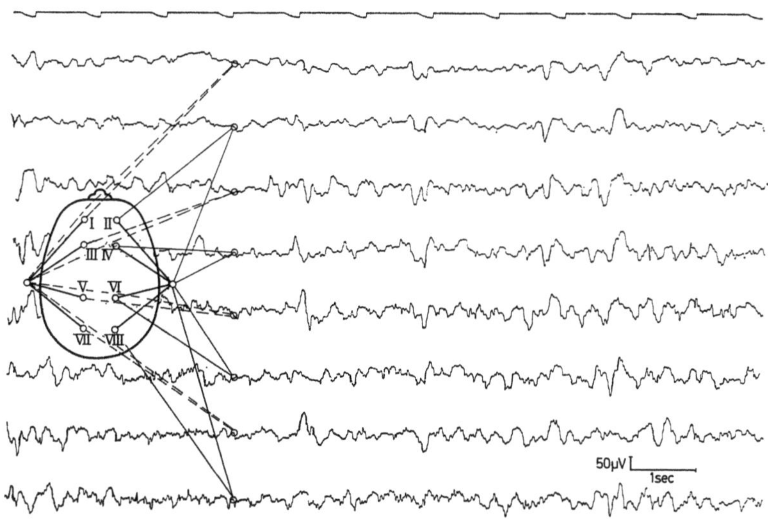

a

July 27, 68

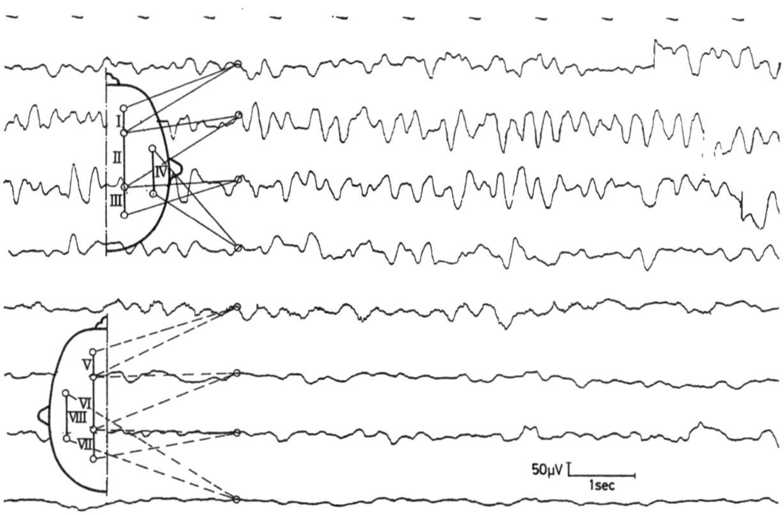

b

Oct. 22, 68

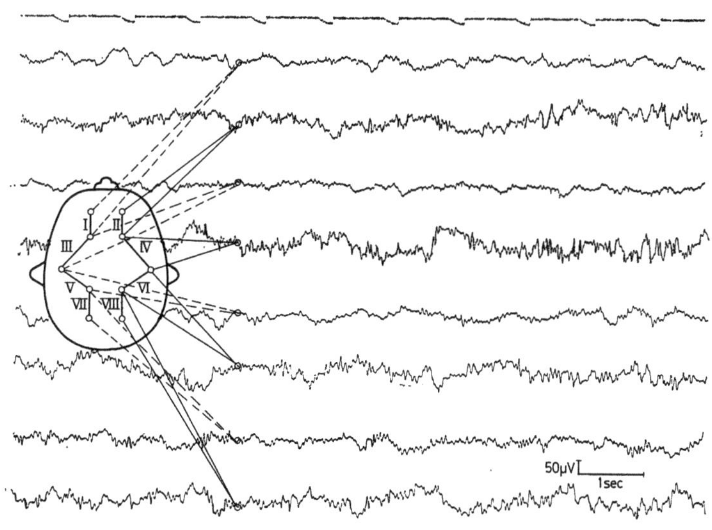

c

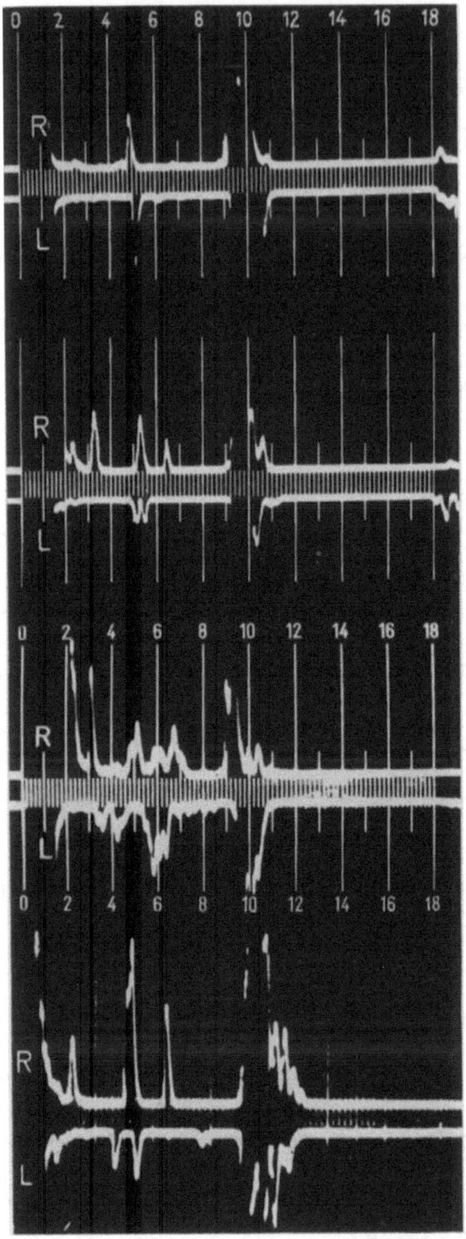

a

b

c

d

Fig. 28 B. Sonoencephalographic follow-up study of the same 5 month old infant (Case No. 2) with multiple congenital defects in partial trisomy D and constitutional thrombopathy with recidivating intracranial hemorrhage. Patient Armin K., SEG No. 1151/69. a) Normal mid-line echo. b) Sonoventriculogram with normal dimensions, although the lateral ventricles are clearly asymmetrical. c) Demonstration of the ventricular system as in b. Definite and strong additional reflections impair the film (hematoma complex). d) Sonoencephalogram after therapy and resorption of the hematoma

SEG: Midline shift absent. Abnormal reflections on the left side (hematoma complex, Fig. 27 a, p. 42).

Clinical Course: The patient expired after 3 days.

Diagnosis: Intracerebral hemorrhage.

Anatomical diagnosis: Intracerebral hemorrhage in the left hemisphere (Fig. 27 b).

Case No. 2

Armin K., 5 months old (File No. 3651). Multiple congenital defects with partial trisomy D were known from the first admission. On July 22, 1968, the patient was readmitted because of repeated tonic, clonic, generalized seizures associated with cyanosis and unconsciousness.

Neurological Status: Alternating convergent strabismus, anisocoria, papilledema; the left pupil was low reacting to light. Opisthotonic posture, facial nerve paresis, and increased patellar reflex on the right side were also present.

Laboratory Findings: Sedimentation rate 13/50, hemoglobin 5 g⁰/₀, erythrocytes 2.22 mil., leucocytes 12,600, thrombocytes 347,000. CSF: xanthochromatic, Pandy's test +, cells 29/3, protein 72 mg-⁰/₀.

Thromboelastogram: Decreased coagulation time, depletion of factor VIII as in constitutional thrombopathy.

EEG: During the first admission on July 1, 1968, a normal EEG was demonstrated with basal activity corresponding to patient age. During the present admission, on July 24., distinct focal alterations in the form of slowing and wave depression over the entire left hemisphere were discovered. The last control before discharge on Aug. 22, demonstrated extensive normalization of the focus (Fig. 28 A, p. 43).

SEG: Sonoencephalographic follow-up studies demonstrated prominent additional reflections (hematoma complex) which were stronger on the left side and corresponded to an intracranial hemorrhage (Fig. 28 B, p. 44). SEG findings were confirmed by further neuroradiological studies.

Diagnosis: Intracerebral hemorrhage in constitutional thrombopathy and multiple congenital defects.

VIII. Sonoencephalographic Examination of Childhood Hydrocephalus

Ultrasonic waves are capable of penetrating the thin cranium of children more easily than when ossification has been completed. Furthermore, when the ventricular system is expanded, it is quite simple to demonstrate the lateral walls of the ventricles on the SEG film. In childhood hydrocephalus, the following measurements can be performed:

a) determination of the width of the lateral ventricles by calculation of the lateral ventricular index,

b) determination of the brain mantle index,

c) determination of the width of the third ventricle,

d) determination of the brain mantle thickness in the fronto-occipital procedure, and

e) determination of the brain mantle thickness in the occipito-frontal procedure.

SEG measurement of the third ventricle and lateral ventricles in childhood was performed for the first time by Lithander in 1961 (see pp. 19, 21). Agreement in SEG values with those obtained from pneumoencephalography has been reported by

SCHIEFER, KAZNER and BRÜCKNER (1963), GELETNEKY and HUMMER (1964), and UMBACH and KLEY (1965). By means of SEG post-operative follow-up studies (after Spitz-Holter oder Pudenz-Heyer drainage), function of the shunt, as demonstrated in decreased or increased ventricular volume, can be closely surveyd.

In all patients referred to our department with signs of hydrocephalus, the following SEG parameters were routinely measured by employing the horizontal beaming technique (Fig. 6): position of the midline echo, width of the lateral ventricles through calculation of the lateral ventricular index, and the width of the third ventricle. As a means of saving film, the lateral ventricular reflections are placed on the upper half and the third ventricle on the lower half of the film (Fig. 13).

Occasionally, reflections originating from the temporal horns can be simultaneously recorded with those from the third ventricle. In cases where simultaneous representation is not possible—this happens more frequently in examining older children—the head of the probe must be slanted at a slightly downward angle (Fig. 16) so that the sonic beam transcends the skull in a slight cranio-caudal direction. From this position, the midline echo and the temporal horn echo can be recorded, so that determination of the brain mantle index is possible (Fig. 24).

In cases of extreme hydrocephalus, determination of the lateral ventricular index is unnecessary, since the bitemporal brain mantle thickness can be measured on the SEG film. This measurement can be directly read from the baseline scale, since the distance between the lateral ventricular echo and the end echo (or initial echo) represents the thickness of the cerebral mantle (Fig. 29). UMBACH and KLEY (1965) recommended measuring the cerebral mantle thickness also in the fronto-occipital and occipito-frontal positions. This form of beaming can only be employed in well-advanced cases of childhood hydrocephalus.

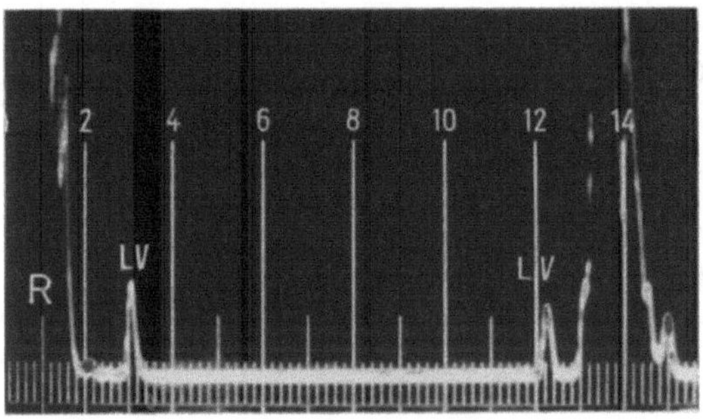

Fig. 29. Sonoencephalogram with extremely expanded lateral ventricles. In this case the brain mantle thickness can be directly determined by measuring the distance between the lateral ventricular wall echo and the end echo respectively in the bitemporal examination

A. Examination of 188 Children with Clinically Suspected Internal Hydrocephalus

We examined 188 children suspected of having internal hydrocephalus of various etiology (Table 7 a). In 14 cases (7.4%) we were unable to determine the lateral ventricular index, and in 67 subjects (35.7%) the brain mantle index was not obtained.

174 patients were divided into the following groups according to lateral ventricular index values: 62 patients (33%) exhibited LVI values within the normal range (< 0.31), 35 (18.6%) revealed values in the border range (LVI = 0.31 ←→ 0.32), and 77 (41%) demonstrated LVIs in the abnormal range (> 0.32). The width of the third ventricle was measured in all 188 subjects, whereby the uppermost borderline for normal values was set a 6 mm. Ninety patients (47.9%) exceeded this border value.

Table 7 a. *Results of SEG examination in 188 cases of suspected hydrocephalus*

Suspected diagnosis	No. of cases	Midline echo shift			Third ventricle			Brain mantle index (BMI)		
Hydrocephalus		under 2 mm	over 2 mm	not measured	normal	over 6 mm	not measured	normal	over 2.3	not measured
LVI not measured	14 (7.4%)	13	1	0	9	5	0	8	6	0
LVI in normal range < 0.31	62 (33%)	61	1	0	59	3	0	25	9	28
LVI in border range 0.31 – 0.32	35 (18.6%)	32	3	0	15	20	0	10	12	13
LVI in abnormal range > 0.32	77 (41%)	67	10	0	15	62	0	0	51	26
Grand total	188	173	15	0	98	90	0	43	78	67
Percentage	100%	92.1	7.9	0	52.1	47.9	0	22.8	41.5	35.7

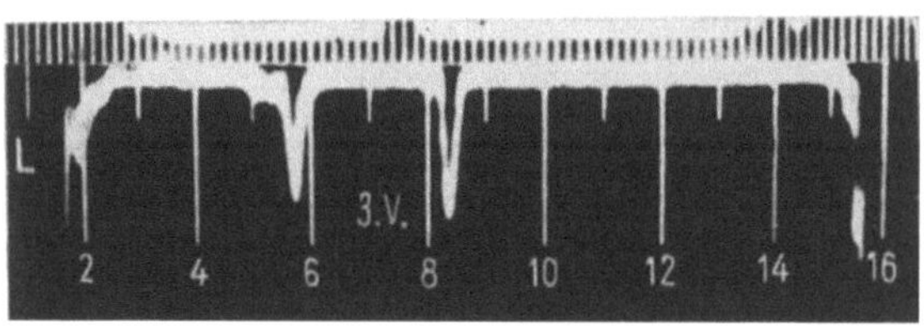

Fig. 30. Sonoencephalogram of a case with an extremely enlarged third ventricle. Third ventricular width is 26 mm

SEG demonstration of the walls of expanded third ventricles is difficult and often unreliable. SCHIEFER and KAZNER obtained SEG measurements of third ventricular dilatation up to 25 – 26 mm, which, according to our experience, seems to be accurate (Fig. 30). PIA and GELETNEKY recommended that the measuring scale be reduced by one-half when third ventricular expansion exceeds 25 mm.

IX. Sonoencephalographic Examination in Intracranial Space-occupying Lesions

In ultrasonic diagnostics of space-occupying cerebral lesions, as well as with other neurological and radiological procedures, the location of the lesions is of great importance. Consequently, the value of the sonoencephalographic examination for diagnosing and localizing space-occupying lesions varies with the position, rate of growth, and type of lesion. The possibilities and limitations of the SEG in diagnosing intracranial tumors through demonstration of tumor echoes has been established by Tanaka, Mitsuno et al. (1956); Wild, Neal, Reid (1950, 1952); Dyk, Barrows and Kruze (1967). Confirming the existence of a space-occupying lesion in vivo in the SEG examination can be established by one of the two methods:

a) direct documentation of reflections originating from the lesion itself, and

b) indirect documentation by demonstration of massive tissue displacement or dilatation of the ventricular system.

The supratentorial hemispheres undergo abnormal tissue displacement as an early sign of expanding neoplastic growth. The extent of accompanying diencephalic midline shift depends on the position and the site of the lesion as well as on coexisting cerebral edema. A unilateral space-occupying lesion in a cerebral hemisphere quickly produces demonstrable tissue displacement, but lesions in the area of the cephalic midline seldom manifest significant SEG shifts.

a) Direct Demonstration

Direct verification of a brain tumor can be established by demonstrating a "tumor-complex" on the oscilloscope screen. In order to directly detect brain tumors by the A-scope method, sufficient ultrasonic reflections and acoustical attenuation are needed. Initial study on this problem was performed by Japanese authors such as Kikuchi and Tanaka et al., and later by Chinese and North American teams such as Walker and Dyk et al. Tanaka et al. consider the following three basic factors necessary for direct SEG confirmation of a cerebral tumor:

1. Shift of the third ventricle or midline echo,
2. Representation of the intracranial tumor echo ("tumor-complex"), and
3. Increased or decreased ultrasonic attenuation.

On the basis of ultrasonic physical findings, Yukishita, Tanaka et al. measured the acoustical impedance of neoplastic tissue and surrounding brain tissue on hand from 62 formalin-fixed preparations (Table 8). The so-called "C-clamp-transducer method" was employed. The authors were also able to determine ultrasonic attenuation of 62 tumors.

According to these examinations, tumor reflections were divided clinically into the following two groups based on their physical characteristics (rate of ultrasonic reflection and acoustical attenuation):

1. Massive tumor echo. a) M-form echo, b) A-form echo.

The M-form echo, which supposedly originates from neoplastic tissue of stronger reflection rates such as meningiomas and craniopharyngiomas, was distinguished by continuous spikes with distinct peaks on both ends.

Table 8. *Acoustical impedance of various types of cerebral tumors as compared to surrounding brain tissue.* (After YUKISHITA et al.)

	No. of cases	Temp. °C	Density (g/cm³)	Sound speed C (cm/sec) $\times 10^5$	Acoustical impedance: Tumor-Tiss. (g/cm²·sec) $\times 10^6$	Acoustical impedance: Surround. Tiss. (g/cm²·sec) $\times 10^6$	Rate of Reflection (%)
Meningioma	15	15	1.061	1.546	0.164	0.157	2.30
Astrocytoma	12	15	1.040	1.503	0.156	0.157	0.58
Glioblastoma m.	7	15	1.041	1.511	0.157	0.157	0.23
Ependymoma	1	15	1.040	1.502	0.156	0.156	0.00
Pinealoma	2	15	1.046	1.507	0.158	0.158	0.16
Medulloblastoma	5	15	1.043	1.497	0.156	0.155	0.58
Oligodendroglioma	1	15	1.042	1.513	0.158	0.159	0.32
Acoust. neurinoma	5	15	1.046	1.491	0.156	0.158	0.83
Craniopharyngioma	2	15	1.050	1.513	0.159	0.156	0.11
Pituit. adenoma	3	15	1.050	1.524	0.159	0.156	1.06
Angioblastoma	1	15	1.044	1.518	0.158	0.159	0.32
Cholesteatoma	1	15	1.044	1.508	0.157	0.157	0.00
Metastat. tumor	7	15	1.044	1.519	0.159	0.157	0.67

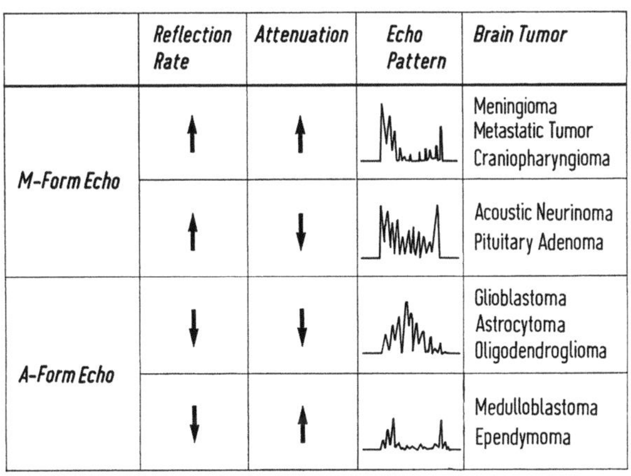

Fig. 31 A. Classification of brain tumor echoes according to their acoustical characteristics. (From YUKISHITA, K., TANAKA, T.: Symposium, Erlangen, West Germany)

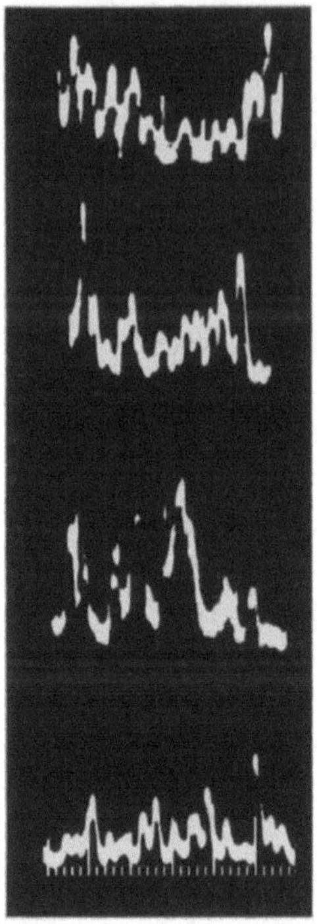

a Craniopharyngioma

b Neurinoma

c Astrocytoma

d Ependymoma

Fig. 31 B. Tumor complex from various brain tumors: a) Craniopharyngioma, SEG No. 1423/70. b) Neurinoma, SEG No. 885/68. c) Astrocytoma, SEG No. 1211/69. d) Ependymoma, SEG No. 965/68. Echo patterns should be compared to Fig. 49 a. By depicting tumor echo patterns, a histological diagnosis can be only suspected

The A-form echo, which supposedly originates from neoplastic tissue of weaker reflection rates, was characterized by an regular undulating base without distinct peaks at the end (Fig. 31 A).

2. Cystic tumor echo. a) macrocystic echo, b) microcystic echo.

This classification is an attempt to clinically differentiate among different types of neoplastic tissue through detailed analysis of the echo pattern originating from the tumor.

We were able to directly detect a tumor complex in 50% of the supratentorial, and 37.5% of the infratentorial confirmed cases.

The physical characteristics of the tumor echoes described by YUKISHITA et al. were compared to those obtained from our patients. As is demonstrated in Fig. 31 B, we were able only to guess at the diagnosis. In accordance with authors such as SCHIEFER, KAZNER, PIA and GELETNEKY, we consider such questionable results somewhat unreliable.

We examined 100 children ranging in age from early infancy to 16 years who were suspected of having an intracranial space-occupying lesion (Table 9).

In 20 patients (20%) the suspicion was verified by SEG and additional neuroradiological methods of examination. An ultrasonic tumor complex was directly

Table 9. *SEG results of 100 patients suspected of possessing an intracranial space-occupying lesion*

Suspected diagnosis	No. of cases	Midline echo displacement (mm)			Lateral ventricular index			Third ventricular width (mm)		
Space-occupying intracranial lesion		under 2	over 2	not measured	normal	over 0.31	not measured	normal	over 7	not measured
Grand total	100	91	9	0	75	17	8	82	14	4
Percentage	100%	91	9	0	75	17	8	82	14	4

demonstrated in 50% of the patients possessing a supratentorial lesion, and in only 37.5% of those patients possessing an infratentorial tumor (Tables 10 and 13). In one case of suspected intracranial space-occupying lesion, we were able to demonstrate an additional echo complex along with a SEG midline shift on the right side. These abnormal reflections were atypical for a tumor complex, since it appeared in the form of a pyramid by weak, as well as increased, sonic wave intensities. It was ultimately proven to be a cerebral abscess (see Case No. 13, Fig. 49 b).

b) Indirect Demonstration

Indirect verification of an intracranial space-occupying lesion can be helpful in establishing early diagnosis. For orientation purposes, these can be divided into the supra and infratentorial lesion.

A. Supratentorial Space-occupying Lesions

The absolutely harmless sonoencephalographic examination renders a great assistance to localizing brain tumors, especially supratentorial tumors. In such cases it is possible that classical clinical symptoms are completely absent. Tonnis and Kränkel were able to demonstrate that out of 1239 patients, only 1/4 of the cases with a tumor located in one of the cerebral hemispheres exhibited papilledema.

Abnormal tissue displacement is the earliest manifestation of a lesion of the supratentorial cerebral hemispheres which can be detected in the SEG. The degree of detectable midline echo shift depends on lesion location and size, as well as on accompanying edema. A unilateral tumor of the cerebral hemispheres produces displacement of midline structures at an early stage. Detectable tissue displacement produced by a space-occupying lesion of the midcephalic area has not been clearly demonstrated in the SEG. We were able to produce SEG verification of mass displacement in 66.7% of the confirmed cases of supratentorial tumors (Table 10). 75% of those exhibited slight to severe ventricular dilatation, and in 50% we were able to demonstrate a tumor complex in the SEG.

Table 10. *Sonoencephalographic and microscopical findings as well as anatomical location of 12 supratentorial mass lesions in children*

Histology of lesion	Location of lesion	Midline echo shift (mm)			Lateral ventricular index			Third ventricle width (mm)			Brain mantle index	Tumor complex
		under 2	over 2	not measured	normal	over 0.31	not measured	normal	over 7	not measured	over 2.3	demonstrated
Glioma	tectum opticum	+	–	–	–	+	–	–	+	–	–	?
Sympatico-blastoma	generalized metastases	+	–	–	+	–	–	+	–	–	–	+
Meningioma	temporal lobe	–	+	–	–	+	–	–	+	–	–	?
Ependymoma	parieto-temporal	–	+	–	–	+	–	–	+	–	–	+
Astrocytoma	temporal lobe	–	+	–	–	+	–	–	+	–	–	+
Astrocytoma	frontal lobe	+	–	–	+	–	–	+	–	–	–	–
Oligodendro-glioma	left hemisphere	–	+	–	–	+	–	+	–	–	–	?
–	in third ventricle	–	+	–	–	+	–	–	–	+	–	?
Ependymoma	basal ganglia	–	+	–	–	+	–	–	+	–	–	+
Abscess	precentral	–	+	–	–	–	+	–	–	+	–	+
–	midbrain	–	+	–	–	+	–	–	–	+	–	?
Craniopharyn-gioma	supra-cellular	+	–	–	–	+	–	–	+	–	–	+
Total	12	4	8	0	2	9	1	3	6	3	0	6
Percent	100	33.3	66.7	0	16	75	12	25	50	25	0	50

B. Infratentorial Space-occupying Lesions

The most frequent tumors of the central nervous system during childhood are located in the infratentorial area. A study of the ratio of infratentorial to supratentorial tumors with advancing age has been made by ANSLING, BAILEY, TÖNNIS and EWERBECK (Table 11).

Infratentorial space-occupying tumors produce enlargement of the ventricular system through occlusion of liquor channels. Depending upon the location of the tumor, one or more portions of the ventricular system can be affected.

Table 11. *Ratio of supratentorial to infratentorial tumors with age.* (After ANSLING et al.)

Age		supratentorial	:	infratentorial
Infancy	– 5 years	1	:	3
5	– 10 years	2	:	3
10	– 15 years	1	:	1
15 years	– adulthood	5	:	1

Table 12. *Indirect SEG findings (midline echo shift and hydrocephalus) according to topographical location of intracranial space-occupying lesion*

			Midline echo shift	Ventricular system dilatation
	Extracerebral	Meninges (unilateral)	+	– –
		Hemispheres (unilateral)	++	– –
	Telencephalon	Lateral ventricles (unilateral)	+	–+
Supratentorial	Suprasellar	Optic nerve	–	–+
		Pituitary	–	–+
		Third ventricle	–	+
		Corpus callosum	–	+
	Midbrain	Septum pellucidum	–	+
		Quadrageminal bodies	–	++
		Pons	– –+	++
	Brainstem	Fourth ventricle	–	++
Infratentorial		Medulla oblongata	–	++
		Hemispheres	–	++
	Cerebellum	Vermis	–	++
		Ponto-cerebellar angle	–	++

Indirect sonoencephalographic findings in supra and infratentorial space-occupying lesions are summarized in Table 12.

We were able to detect only 8 infratentorial tumors with the SEG (Table 13). The majority were children under 5 years of age. In only two cases (12.5%) could abnormal tissue displacement be demonstrated, but all patients exhibited accompany-

Table 13. *SEG, microscopical and anatomical findings in 8 cases of infratentorial tumors*

Anatomical location	Histology	Midline echo shift (mm)			Lateral ventricular index			Third ventricular width (mm)			BMI	Tumor complex
		under 2	over 2	not measured	normal	over 0.31	not measured	normal	over 7	not measured	over 2.3	demonstrated
Pons	—	—	+	—	—	+	—	—	+	—	—	?
Pons	—	—	+	—	—	+	—	—	+	—	—	?
Pons	Glio-blastoma	+	—	—	—	+	—	—	+	—	—	+
Pons	Astro-cytoma	+	—	—	—	+	—	—	+	—	—	+
Pons	—	+	—	—	—	+	—	—	+	—	+	?
Cerebellar Vermis	Spongio-blastoma	+	—	—	—	+	—	—	+	—	+	?
Cerebellum	Medullo-blastoma	+	—	—	—	+	—	—	+	—	—	—
Cerebellum	Ependymoma	+	—	—	—	+	—	—	+	—	—	+
Total	8	6	2	0	0	8	0	0	8	0	2	3
Percent	100%	75	25	0	0	100	0	0	100	0	25	37.5

ing ventricular dilatation. Additional reflections which could definitely be contributed to the tumor were found in only 3 (37.5%) of the patients.

In summary, it must be stressed that early manifestations of intracranial lesions can be indirectly detected in the sonoencephalogram by demonstration of hydrocephalus or midline echo shifts, which also enable lateral localization of the lesion. A definite histological diagnosis should not be attempted. Neither does a normal SEG eliminate the possibility of an intracranial space-occupying lesion (Fig. 52 b). In such cases, a combined SEG-EEG examination usually enables a general diagnosis to be established (see Chapter XIV).

X. Congenital and Developmental Defects and Brain Damage in Early Childhood

A number of neurological-psychiatric disease entities, e. g., cerebral palsy, are usually the result of brain damage in early childhood and do not necessarily represent uniform denotation in their clinical symptoms, etiology or morphology. In order to classify brain damage during early childhood, one must consider the moment of the noxious influence, the etiology, anatomical location of the damage and clinical symptoms. However, classification based on the moment of damage occurrence has proven useful. This can be divided accordingly into the following three groups:

a) the intrauterine and prenatal period,

b) the perinatal period, and

c) the postnatal period.

Traumas and noxious influences during early childhood cause brain damage with manifold clinical symptoms. All brain damage that affects the immature brain and leads to defects in cerebral structures falls into the category of *infantile encephalopathy*. Moreover, one must include in this group all prenatal, natal and postnatal damage, since development of the cerebrum extends into the fourth year of life. Usually such damage is secondary to congenital central nervous system defects, perinatal anoxia, hemorrhage, metabolic disorders, perinatal or postnatal infections, or trauma (PIA, GELETNEKY).

A. Sonoencephalographic Findings

Localized and diffuse cerebral atrophy, as well as cystic changes, offer good conditions for SEG examination; namely, through additional reflections which originate from interfaces of abnormal structures. These are easily demonstrable in children, due to the thin boney structures of the immature cranium.

In the group of infantile encephalopathies, the following SEG changes can be observed:

1. displacement of the midline structures,
2. enlargement of the ventricular system, and
3. additional reflections.

Displacement of midline structures is produced by atrophy of a hemisphere, which can be detected in the SEG by a midline echo shift toward the affected side. Also, atrophical *enlargement of the ventricles* can be detected and evaluated by calculation of the lateral ventricular index and determination of third ventricular width. GELETNEKY (1965, 1966) interpreted *additional reflections* (wall-echoes) and echo-free zones as cystic changes. Furthermore, he observed shifts of the midline echo in 11 of 14 cases with unilateral cerebral atrophy.

Correct interpretation of cystic wall-echoes that appear in various birth defects and porencephaly is difficult and requires considerable experience. SCHIEFER and KAZNER demonstrated enlargement of the ventricles and cystic changes resulting from earlier cerebral damage not only in children, but also in adults.

We examined 90 children which were categorized into one of the following groups according to preliminary clinical examinations: atrophical and cystic changes, congenital birth defects of the brain and/or retarded psychomotoric development, and cerebral damage during early childhood (Table 14).

In 9 cases (10%) abnormal displacement of the midline echo toward the affected side could be demonstrated. In each of these cases neuroradiological documentation of the shift was possible. An example is presented in Case No. 10.

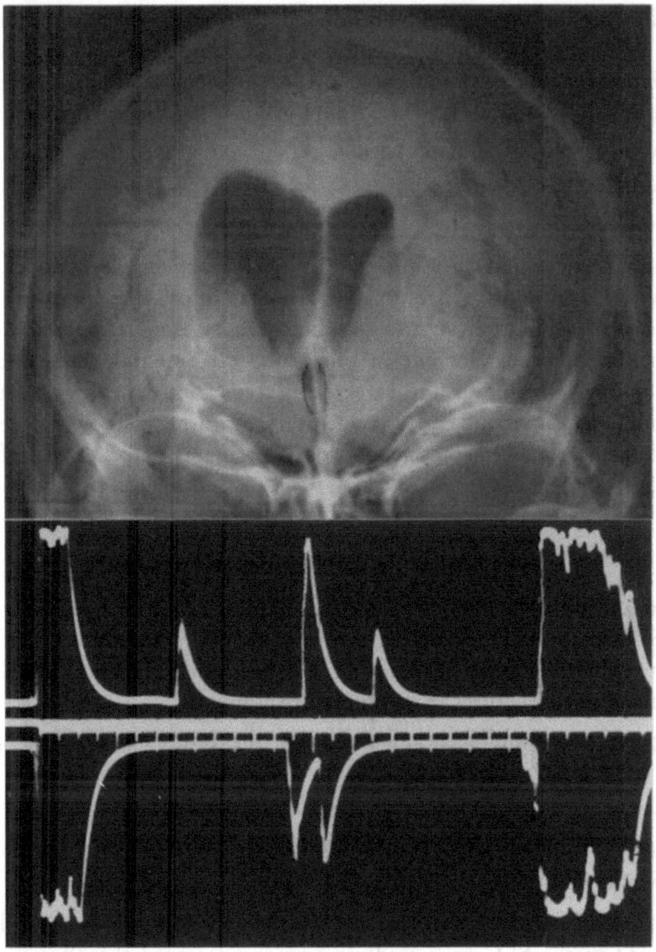

Fig. 32. Sonoencephalogram and air encephalogram of a child with asymmetrical dilatation of the lateral ventricles resulting from perinatal cerebral damage. Complete correlation can be observed

Ventricular enlargement, varying from symmetrical to asymmetrical dilatation (Fig. 32), which was attributed to one of the infantile encephalopathies, was demonstrated in 23 subjects (Table 14). A one-year old child exhibited not only an enlarged ventricular system (Fig. 33), but also a positive diaphane. Consequently, we were able to make a preliminary diagnosis of the Dandy-Walker syndrome, which was confirmed by a later PEG examination.

Additional reflections could be demonstrated in the sonoencephalogram of only 3 patients (3.3%) included in Table 14 (Fig. 48 b). An example is presented in Case No. 12.

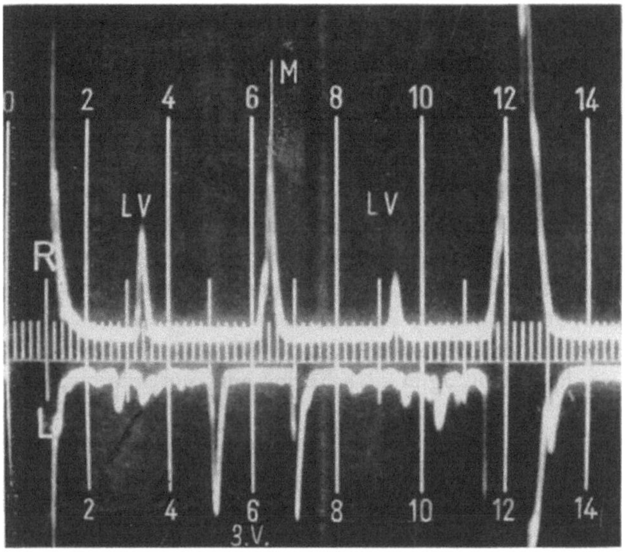

Fig. 33. Abnormal sonoencephalogram of a one-year old child with Dandy-Walker syndrome (SEG No. 649/68). Lateral ventricular index = $\frac{60}{117+6}$ = 0.48. Third ventricular width = 20 mm

Table 14. *SEG findings in 90 children with damage to the brain*

Suspected diagnosis	No. of cases	Midline echo shift			Lateral ventricular index			Third ventricle			Brain mantle index			Additional reflections (cystic echoes)
Infantile encephalopathy		under 2 mm	over 2 mm	not measured	under 0.31 normal	over 0.31	not measured	normal	pathological	not measured	normal	over 2.3	not measured	
Atrophy and cystic changes	7	4	3	0	3	3	1	5	2	0	0	1	6	1
Congenital and developmental defect	64	59	5	0	48	15	1	56	8	0	32	12	20	2
Cerebral damage in early childhood	19	18	1	0	14	5	0	17	2	0	3	6	10	0
Grand total	90	81	9	0	65	23	2	78	12	0	35	19	36	3
Percent	100	90	10	0	71	26	3	87	13	0	39	21	40	3.3

B. Prenatally Determined Brain Damage as Sometimes Exhibited in Phenylketonuria

SEG Examination of Cerebral Atrophy in 31 Treated and 14 Untreated PKU Patients

The pathological entity of phenylketonuria (PKU), which was originally described by FØLLING in 1934, is attributed to an inborn error of protein metabolism. The primary metabolic abnormality is the inherited deficiency of the liver enzyme phenylalanin-4-hydroxylase. The clinical manifestations are severe mental retardation with multiple neurological signs. A number of review articles such as those of MAUTNER and QUINN; JERVIS, PAIN, WRIGHT and TARJANA; and LANG have emphasized the combination of a severe mental defect and micrencephaly with blue eyes, blond hair, light skin, agitated behavior and, not infrequently, epilepsy and eczema.

A morphological examination of the cerebral structures of phenylketonurics was performed for the first time by ALVORD et al. who described an alteration of the myelin structures. BENDA, CORSELLIS, JERVIS, SCHOLZ, POSER and VAN BOGAERT; CROME and PARE; and MALAMUD reported the post-mortem findings from PKU patients of various ages and were able to observe inconstant changes of arrested myelination and/or demyelination in the form of pallor or spongy foci in the white matter. The demyelination was combined with a corresponding mild or intensive gliosis. These alterations appear to be a major factor for the presence of micrencephaly in PKU.

Macroscopical observations of cerebral atrophy have included diminished brain mass with reduced weight, mild convolutional anomalies, dilatation of the ventricles and subarachnoideal space, and in one case, porencephaly. BECHER et al. reported a case of phenylketonuria exhibiting an intermittent progressive course. BICKEL, GRÜTER, and MALAMUD suggested a correlation between the clinical course and the neuropathological findings. MALAMUD emphasized that while the spongy lesions were the exclusive changes in younger patients, demyelinating lesions became manifest only at a more advanced age, where they appeared to be superimposed on an earlier spongy change.

Cerebral atrophy can be detected in clinical examination by several methods. Whereas many authors have described various functional abnormalities in phenylketonuria in the form of EEG alterations, only a few pneumoencephalographic studies have been carried out. Dilatation of the ventricles and enlargement of the subarachnoideal space was first demonstrated in the pneumoencephalogram by JERVIS. MAUTNER and QUINN also reported pathological PEG findings in PKU. The most complete study to date was done by SUFFCZYNSKA-KOTOWSKA et al., who were able to evaluate the pneumoencephalograms in 11 out of 12 PKU patients. They observed cerebral atrophy in 8 cases, varying from symmetrical or asymmetrical ventricular dilatation to reduction of the cerebral cortex, with corresponding enlargement of the gyri, and in one case, porencephaly.

We examined 45 patients with confirmed phenylketonuria. They were divided into the following groups:

Group 1 consisted of 31 children, aged 3 months to 8 years 3 months, currently undergoing dietary treatment at the Heidelberg University Children's Hospital. The diagnosis was established by Guthrie-test, column or thin-layer chromatography of the blood, and by the $FeCl_3$-test and chromatographic analysis of the urine. The time of initiation of dietary treatment varied from the first week post-partum to 3½ years of age (see Table 15 for details).

Group 2 consisted of 14 patients from the Johannes-Anstalten Mosbach*, ranging in age from 9¾ to 37¾ years (see Table 16). These patients were diagnosed as phenylketonurics on the basis of Guthrie-test, column chromatography and $FeCl_3$-test.

All sonoencephalographic examinations were performed according to procedure described in Chapter V.

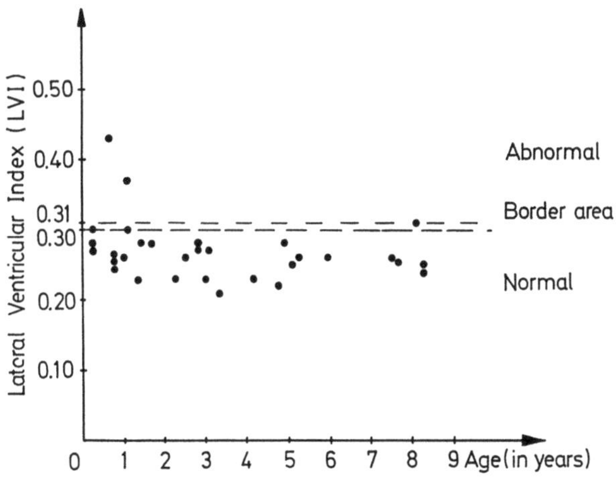

Fig. 34 a. Graphical representation of the lateral ventricular indices of 31 dietetically treated phenylketonurics. Only 2 patients demonstrated abnormal values—a further 3 were found to have LVIs in the upper border

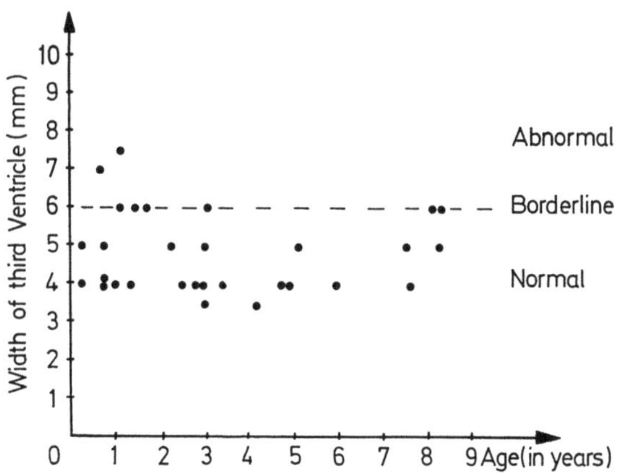

Fig. 34 b. Graphical representation of SEG values for third ventricular width in 31 dietetically treated phenylketonurics. Only 2 children demonstrated abnormal values of 7 and 8 mm, all others being within normal range

* Acknowledgements are made to Dr. ENGLER, the director of this hospital, and his staff for making this study possible.

From the data in Table 15 the following observations can be made:

1. From 31 dietetically treated patients, 2 exhibited abnormally large lateral ventricular indices. Three patients were found to be in the border value range, and the remaining 26 displayed normal lateral ventricles (Fig. 34 a).

2. In 2 cases the third ventricle was found to be abnormally dilated to 7 and 8 mm, while the remaining 29 patients showed normal values (Fig. 34 b).

3. A midline echo shift, expressing displacement of tissue masses, could not be found in any of these patients.

Table 15. *Sonoencephalographic and clinical data on 31 dietetically treated PKU children*

Name	Age (years)	SEG-Number	Time span from birth to initiation of diet	IQ or DQ	Seizures	Lateral ventricular index (LVI)	Third ventricle (mm)	Midline echo shift (mm)
Ines K.	$3^5/_{12}$	1429/70	1 week	IQ= 115	—	0.21	4	0
Petra J.	$1^1/_{12}$	1501/70	1 week	DQ= 97	—	0.37	7–8	0
Petra M.	$^1/_4$	1367/70	1 week	DQ= 86	—	0.30	5	1
Michael W.	$^2/_3$	1500/70	2 weeks	DQ= 99	—	0.43	7	0
Manuela B.	$^3/_4$	1446/70	2 weeks	DQ= 92	—	0.25	4	1
Gesine H.	$^3/_4$	1223/69	2 weeks	DQ= 98	—	0.25	4	0.5
Wolfgang S.	$^1/_4$	1350/70	2 weeks	DQ= 108	—	0.28	5	0
Michael F.	$1^1/_{12}$	1349/70	2 weeks	DQ= 90	—	0.30	6	1.5
Klaus-P. F.	$^1/_4$	1186/69	3 weeks	DQ= 93	—	0.28	4	0
Susanne K.	$2^5/_6$	1207/69	3 weeks	DQ= 107	—	0.24	4	0
Axel B.	$4^3/_4$	1248/69	4 weeks	IQ= 116	—	0.22	4	1
Marko K.	$^3/_4$	1420/70	4 weeks	IQ= 107	—	0.26	5	2
René M.	$5^1/_4$	1260/69	5 weeks	IQ= 112	—	0.26	4.5	1
Christiane S.	$7^1/_2$	1251/69	2 months	IQ= 110	—	0.23	4	0.5
Monika K.	$2^5/_6$	1316/69	2 months	DQ= 90	—	0.28	6	0

Table 15 (continued)

Name	Age (years)	SEG-Number	Time span from birth to initiation of diet	IQ or DQ	Seizures	Lateral ventricular index (LVI)	Third ventricle (mm)	Midline echo shift (mm)
Friedrich H.	$8^{1}/_{4}$	1249/69	2 months	IQ= 95	–	0.24	5	0.5
Manuela G.	$4^{1}/_{6}$	1250/69	2 months	IQ= 110	–	0.23	4	0
Sabine D.	$1^{1}/_{3}$	1224/69	3 months	DQ= 88	–	0.23	4	0.5
Markus T.	$2^{1}/_{4}$	1307/69	6 months	DQ= 64	–	0.28	5	0.5
Sabine B.	$4^{11}/_{12}$	1512/70	6 months	IQ= 93	+	0.28	4	0
Jörg Sch.	1	1145/69	10 months	DQ= 72	–	0.26	4	0
Wolfgang M.	$2^{1}/_{2}$	1216/69	10 months	DQ= 61	+	0.26	4	0.5
Susanne W.	$1^{5}/_{12}$	1487/70	$1^{1}/_{6}$ years	DQ= 80	–	0.28	6	1.5
Horst Sch.	$8^{1}/_{2}$	1121/69	$1^{1}/_{3}$ years	IQ= 36	+	0.31	6	0
Oliver Sch.	$1^{2}/_{3}$	1499/70	$1^{1}/_{3}$ years	DQ= 64	–	0.28	6	0
Olaf K.	3	1188/69	$1^{5}/_{12}$ years	DQ= 89	–	0.23	3.5	0
Alexandra K.	$3^{1}/_{12}$	1509/70	2 years	DQ= 49	+	0.27	6	0
Gabriela G.	$8^{1}/_{4}$	1121/69	$2^{1}/_{3}$ years	DQ= 37	++	0.25	6	1
Thomas K.	$5^{1}/_{12}$	1352/69	$2^{5}/_{6}$ years	DQ= 63	–	0.25	5	0
Stefan Sch.	$7^{1}/_{2}$	1416/70	$3^{3}/_{4}$ years	IQ= 73	–	0.26	5	0
Thomas K.	$5^{11}/_{12}$	1242/69	$3^{3}/_{4}$ years	IQ= 80	+	0.26	4	0.5

4. The development quotient (DQ), which was measured by the Bühler/Hetzer-Kleinkindertest (analogue to Gesell test) in those between 0 to 3 years of age, and the intelligence quotients (IQ), which was measured by the Binet/Kramertest (analogue to Stanfort-Binet) in those patients over 3 years of age, varied from 36 to 116. A statistically valid correlation between age of diet initiation and intelligence level can be demonstrated in our group (Kaiser and Bickel, 1969).

5. Six patients were reported to have had a history of seizures.

6% (2 patients) of the dietetically treated group exhibited cerebral atrophy in the form of pronounced dilatation of the ventricular system. It is interesting to note that both of these individuals experienced complications during birth.

In Table 16 the measured values for the untreated group are recorded as follows:

1. From a total of 14 patients, 10 exhibited a LVI larger than 0.31, therefore distinctively abnormal. Two displayed border range values, and only two were within normal limits (Fig. 35 a).

2. In 10 cases the third ventricle was dilated from 6.5 to 9 mm, thereby indicating atrophy. In 3 patients the diameter of the third ventricle was measured to be

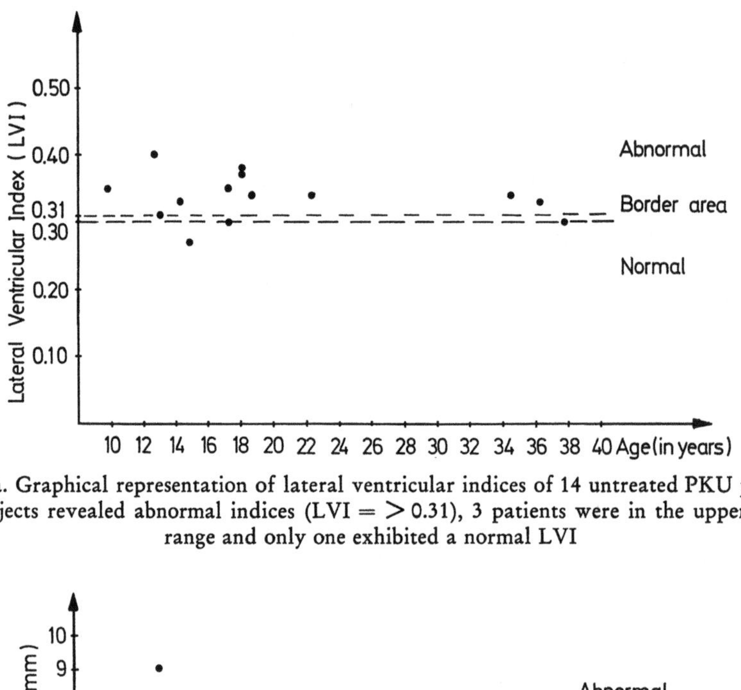

Fig. 35 a. Graphical representation of lateral ventricular indices of 14 untreated PKU patients. Ten subjects revealed abnormal indices (LVI = > 0.31), 3 patients were in the upper border range and only one exhibited a normal LVI

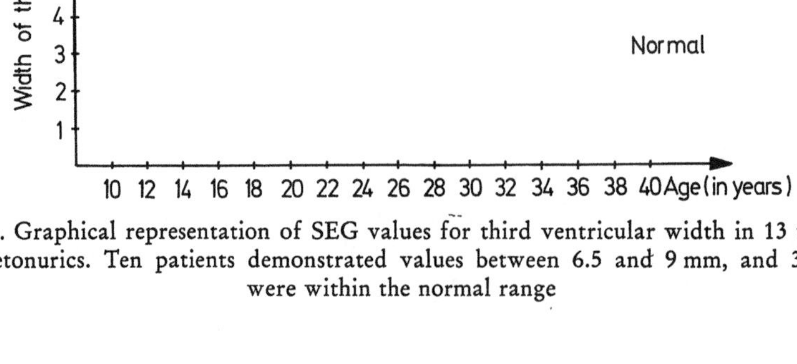

Fig. 35 b. Graphical representation of SEG values for third ventricular width in 13 untreated phenylketonurics. Ten patients demonstrated values between 6.5 and 9 mm, and 3 patients were within the normal range

Table 16. *Sonoencephalographic and clinical data on 14 untreated youths and adult PKU patients*

Name	Age (years)	SEG-Number	Intel-ligence level	Sei-zures	Lateral ventri-cular index (LVI)	Third ven-tricle (mm)	Mid-line echo shift (mm)
Norma W.	$9^3/_4$	1411/70	idiot	+	0.35	8	0
Sabine E.	$12^2/_3$	1407/70	imbecile	—	0.40	—	0
Karl-H. W.	$13^1/_{12}$	1409/70	idiot	—	0.31	9	0
Mercedes H.	$14^1/_3$	1412/70	imbecile	—	0.33	6—6.5	—
Fred G.	$14^{11}/_{12}$	1406/70	idiot	—	0.27	6	0
Uwe S.	$17^1/_3$	1410/70	imbecile	—	0.35	6	0.5
Bruno C.	$17^5/_{12}$	1403/70	imbecile	—	0.30	8—8.5	3
Erwin H.	$18^1/_{12}$	1401/70	idiot	—	0.37	7	1
Wilfred H.	$18^1/_{12}$	1402/70	idiot	—	0.38	8	0
Siegfried K.	$18^2/_3$	1408/70	imbecile	—	0.34	7.5	1.5
Johanna M.	$22^1/_3$	1399/70	idiot	—	0.34	7.5	2
Manfred W.	$34^1/_4$	1398/70	imbecile	—	0.34	6	1
Horst R.	$36^1/_6$	1405/70	idiot	—	0.33	8	0.5
Martin W.	$37^3/_4$	1404/70	idiot	—	0.30	8	0

6 mm, representing the upper normal value, and in one patient the third ventricle could not be determined (Fig. 35 b).

3. Clear representation of the midline reflections of one subject was not possible. An abnormal shift of the midline echo of 3 mm toward the right occurred in one case. Further EEG studies revealed a focus of delta wave activity over the right hemisphere extending from the frontal precentral area to the temporal area. Since both EEG focus and SEG shift were demonstrated on the right side, unilateral atrophy of the right hemisphere can be assumed.

4. All the patients of this group were found to be imbecile or idiotic.

5. Two 18 year old patients of this group were monozygotic twins, both exhibiting severe mental deficiency, analogous laboratory findings, and pronounced cerebral atrophy as expressed in similar SEG findings.

6. A history of local convulsions could be obtained in one case. These extended mainly over a period of 3 months.

92.8% (13 patients) of the untreated group exhibited cerebral atrophy in the form of a pronounced ventricular dilatation. 50% demonstrated an enlargement of all components of the ventricular system, 21.4% (3 cases) displayed isolated third ventricular dilatation, and 21.4% (3 cases) revealed isolated lateral ventricular enlargement.

The morphological basis and the onset of cerebral damage varies in different inborn metabolic diseases, and is in numerous aspects as yet unclear. A diffuse inhibition of myelination is generally observed in PKU, which, according to GRÜTER, is chronologically correlated with the development of mental deficiency. Corresponding to the disturbed myelination, the PKU patient develops a progredient mental defect during early childhood, which proceeds to a more stationary phase after puberty. Exceptions have been reported. Perry et al. have suggested that a chronic insufficiency of glutamine, found only in PKU patients with severe mental defects, may play a part in damaging the growing human brain.

In our study of 14 untreated adolescent and adult phenylketonurics who presented the classical picture of PKU, 13 (92.8%) exhibited cerebral atrophy in the form of abnormal ventricular expansion. In the group of 31 dietetically treated children, however, only 2 cases (6%) exhibited marked cerebral atrophy. The clinical manifestations observed in the treated group were manifold: several children had convulsions; the IQ and phenylalanine blood levels before the dietary treatment were varied and showed no correlation. A comparison of the two groups indicates that a correlation between cerebral atrophy and intelligence exists in the advanced phase of PKU. Stadler found in his examination of 9 PKU patients ranging in age from 4 to 13 years, a relatively good correlation between the degree of EEG anomalies, PEG changes, and mental deficiency. The cerebral atrophy observed in our cases cannot be attributed to ictal damage, since, in those patients exhibiting a pathological ventricular enlargement, no chronic convulsive disorders or status epilepticus were known.

The extent to which cerebral atrophy in PKU is finally inhibited by dietary treatments remains to be answered by future investigations.

XI. Sonoencephalographic Examination in Various Convulsive Disorders

The primary value of the SEG examination in the presence of epilepsy should be to determine whether the condition is secondary to cerebral damage or is of non-organic origin. The most frequent causes of childhood epilepsy are trauma, infection, congenital and metabolic defects, and cerebral hypoxia.

Space-occupying lesions, scars, and other localized cerebral damage can give rise to focal or generalized convulsive disorders. Early detection of the lesions is of primary importance in correct diagnosis and therapy.

In this manner, the SEG can often render a useful service and, at times, establish complete clarification of the case.

We examined 139 children with convulsive seizures of various etiologies (Table 17 a). Fourty-eight subjects (34.5%) exhibited enlarged lateral ventricles of which 3 were found to be asymmetrically dilated. Fourty patients (28.8%) displayed third ventricular enlargement, and an abnormal midline echo shift was detected in 2 cases. The cause of the displaced tissue masses was determined in combination with EEG examinations (see Case No. 10 and 12, Chapter XIV). Further SEG studies were performed on 26 children with infectious seizures (Table 17 b). Abnormal expansion of the lateral ventricles and of the third ventricle was demonstrated in 6 subjects (23.1%).

In this manner, the SEG enables quick orientation concerning the position of the hemispheres, atrophical changes, ventricular dilatation, and possible asymmetry. Rapid orientation as to the degree of organic brain damage in the epileptic patient can possibly be determined.

Table 17 a. *Results of sonoencephalographic examination of 139 children with petit and grand mal seizures of various etiology*

Diagnosis	Number of cases	Midline echo shift			Lateral ventricular index (LVI)			Third ventricle			Brain mantle index (BMI)		
Seizures (petit and grand mal) of various etiology		under 2 mm	over 2 mm	not measured	under 0.30	over 0.30	not measured	under 6 mm	over 6 mm	not measured	under 2.3	over 2.3	not measured
Total No.	139	137	2	0	89	48	2	99	40	0	88	41	10
Percent	100	98.6	1.4	0	64	34.5	1.5	71.2	28.8	0	63.3	29.5	7.2

Table 17 b. *Results of sonoencephalographic examination of 26 children with infectious seizures*

Diagnosis	No. of cases	Midline echo shift			Lateral ventricular index (LVI)			Third ventricle			Brain mantle index (BMI)		
Infectious seizures		under 2 mm	over 2 mm	not measured	under 0.30	over 0.30	not measured	under 6 mm	over 6 mm	not measured	under 2.3	over 2.3	not measured
Total No.	26	26	0	0	19	6	1	20	6	0	14	5	7
Percent	100	100	0	0	73.1	23.1	3.8	76.9	23.1	0	53.9	19.2	26.9

When SEG results in epileptics are compared to those obtained by the pneumoencephalogram, the absolute number of abnormal findings in the PEG can be expected to be larger.

Air encephalographic studies in childhood convulsive disorders have been reported by several authors. BAMBERGER and MATTHES demonstrated pathological PEG findings in 62%, and SHATVEDT et al. in 60% of their series of children with seizures.

BAMBERGER and MATTHES (1959) performed PEG examinations in 137 children with convulsive disorders and reported the following results: 49 children exhibited normal ventricular parameters, 41 demonstrated symmetrical dilatation, and 41 asymmetrical dilatation. Six congenital developmental defects were discovered. SHATVEDT et al. demonstrated abnormal PEGs in 60% of 165 patients with convulsive attacks.

However, as a preliminary orientation procedure, the SEG's purpose is to indicate the need for a pneumoencephalogram, as well as to perform follow-up studies. In addition, it is valuable in detecting ictal changes.

XII. Reliability of the Sonoencephalogram in the Diagnosis of Childhood Hydrocephalus

Evaluation of cerebral structures, especially appraisal of the ventricular system, is of great importance in pediatrics. Early diagnosis of childhood hydrocephalus and prompt initiation of therapy are decisive in the prognosis of this disorder.

In every case of macrocephalus or suspected increased intracranial pressure, it is infeasible to perform a pneumoencephalogram, since this examination represents a major procedure, in which complications can arise. Therefore, the usual course before pneumoencephalography has been to graphically follow the circumference of the skull and to observe other clinical signs of increased pressure. Sonoencephalography has provided a means of obtaining this information in pediatric diagnostics.

The reliability in determination of the midline echo has been examined by authors such as DEVLIEGER, RIDDLER, FORD and AMBROSE; JEFFERSON, JEPPSON, TAYLOR et al.; SCHIEFER and KAZNER; and WHITE. They reported statistical validity in 92 to 98% of their cases. In PEG-SEG examinations of normal third ventricles by JACOBI and SCHUCH; FEUERLEIN et al.; FORD and MCRAE; UEMATSU (1966); SJÖGREN, WEST, and MOSTAFAWY (1969), agreement was found in 90 to 99% of the cases. In abnormal cases with mass tissue displacement, the quota decreased to 24.7% (SCHIEFER and KAZNER).

PEG-SEG agreement in measurement of the width of the lateral ventricles was reported by several of the above-mentioned authors.

Reliability of the SEG in the diagnosis of childhood hydrocephalus as compared to pneumoencephalographic values and other clinical data will be dealt with in the following chapter.

Subject Matter

The following study consists of 110 patients ranging in age from 3 months to 12 years in whom 243 SEG examinations were carried out. Table 18 gives the distribution of the various age groups.

Table 18. *Age distribution of 110 children suspected of/or having hydrocephalus*

Age (in years)	No. of cases
< 1	33
1 to 4	42
5 to 10	27
11 to 13	8
	110

All of the 110 children were referred to our department either because of suspected hydrocephalus or because an enlarged ventricular system was discovered during routine examination. In 60 of the 110 children a follow-up air encephalogram was performed after SEG examination. Consequently, we were able to evaluate combined SEG-PEG findings in order to judge the reliability of SEG representation of the ventricular system. So that SEG results of the remaining 50 children (in whom a

PEG was not made) could be critically evaluated, an appraisal of the correlation between SEG and clinical data was undertaken. The examinations were performed with a SEG Siemens apparatus (after Krautkrämer), and with a SEG apparatus by Kretz-Technik (series 4100 ME) (Fig. 4). After measurement of the bitemporal cranial diameter with callipers, the examination was performed in the usual manner.

The probe is suffused with a transmission substance and placed horizontally on the squamous portion of the temporal bone above the external auditory meatus (Fig. 6). From a distance of 2 to 4 cm above the ear, orientation of the midline structure is accomplished by identifying reflections originating from the septum pellucidum from both sides of the skull. A search is then made for reflections from the outer walls of the third ventricle. In our experience with children, we have found that the external probe position in the pediatric examination lies somewhat posterior to that used in the adult examination, i. e., directly above the ear. Next, the lateral ventricles and the falx cerebri are demonstrated from a position on the upper portion of the temporal bone (Fig. 6 and 7). Reflections from both planes originating from the outer walls of the lateral ventricles are captured on the SEG film (Fig. 36 a). It has proven practical to place the lateral ventricular echoes on the upper half of the SEG film and the third ventricular echoes on the lower half. This cor-

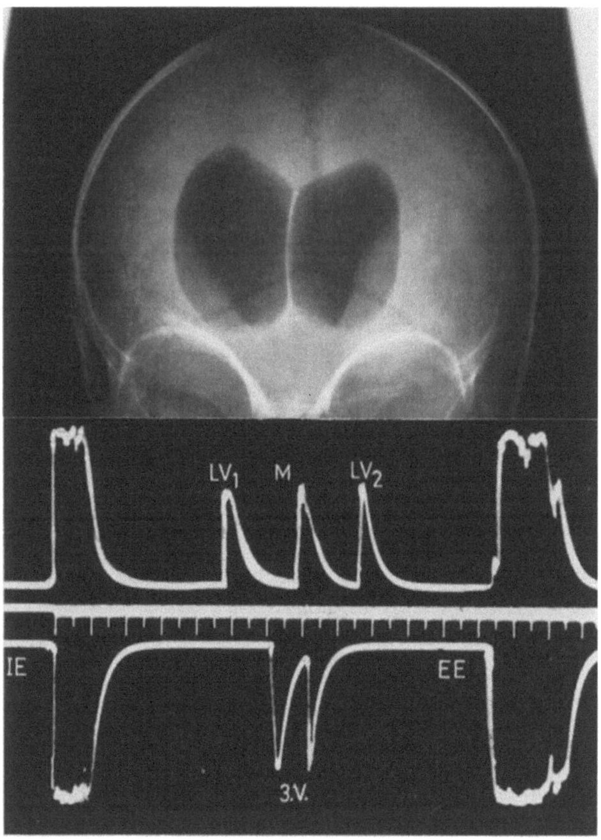

Fig. 36 a. Sonoencephalogram and pneumoencephalogram of infant with an abnormal ventricular system. SEG apparatus from Kretz-Technik, series 4100 ME. Abb.: LV_1 and LV_2 = outer wall of the lateral ventricles, 3.V. = third ventricle, M = midline echo

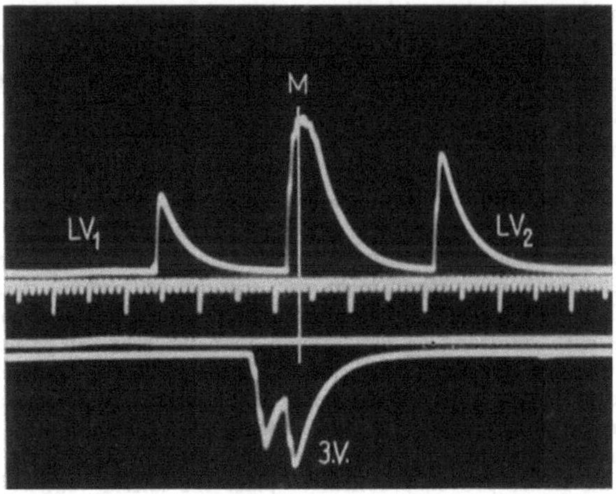

Fig. 36 b. Taken from Fig. 36 a. By means of an electronic magnifier, midline structures can be enlarged on the oscilloscope screen. Distances can be more exactly determined. Abb.: LV_1 and LV_2 = outer walls of the lateral ventricles, 3.V. = third ventricle, M = midline echo

responds to true anatomical relationships. In some cases we used electronic magnification to enlarge the middle portion of the screen, since this made evaluation of the film easier (Fig. 36 b).

A. Comparison of SEG Results with Other Clinical Data

a) Examination

The results of our SEG examination of 50 children and the pertinent clinical observations, such as notable cranial growth, macrocephalus with and without progression, and signs of increased cerebral pressure are compared in Table 19. A + indicates that significant results were demonstrated, a – represents insignificant results, and a ○ signifies that we were unable to make a statement in this case. We outlined our SEG results in the following 5 categories:

1 a) *Width of the third ventricle.* For evaluation purposes we referred to our normal values in healthy children with the uppermost border of the norm set at 6 mm (see p. 20).

1 b) When the *lateral ventricular index* exceeded 0.32, we concluded that an abnormal dilatation existed (see pp. 25, 30, 76).

1 c) We referred to an *increase in ventricular width* when at least two SEG control examinations demonstrated progressive intensification.

1 d) Determination of *brain mantle thickness* is significant in extreme hydrocephalus. Isolated peripheral reflections originating from the lateral ventricles are not easily differentiated from temporal horn reflections. In such cases, delineation of the midline echo is not always possible. Consequently, determination of the lateral ventricular index or the brain mantle index is unnecessary (Fig. 29). A brain mantle thickness under 2 cm can be confirmed by positive transillumination.

Transillumination or diaphane is a method in which an examination lamp is placed on the cranium of the patient in complete darkness. Lateral reflection of light rays is hindered by a firm rubber cuff. When the brain mantle thickness is less than 1.5 to 2.0 cm, the cranial vault is illuminated in an abnormally enlarged area. This method is most frequently employed in the detection of subdural hygromas.

1 e) The fifth category can be divided into the "*normal ventricular system*", and "*ventricular system in the borderline area*". The borderline area is composed of lateral ventricular indices between 0.30 and 0.32. Values in this category require additional data in order to verify whether a normal or an enlarged ventricular system exists.

The clinical data which point to the existence of hydrocephalus are comprised of the following 8 criteria:

1 f) *Confirmed hydrocephalus* diagnosed by earlier clinical examination, e. g., PEG.

1 g) *Noticeable increase in cranial circumference.* Macrocephalus with or without progressive growth was the most frequent observation.

1 h) *Transillumination* enabled confirmation in many cases where the brain mantle thickness was less than 2 cm.

1 i) *Signs of increased intracranial pressure* (such as papilledema, headache, and tense fontanelles) were considered important indications of hydrocephalus.

1 j) *Cerebral damage in early childhood and retardation of psychomotoric development* was usually present when the SEG demonstrated enlargement of the ventricles and additional reflections, without the pre-existence of any of the above clinical signs.

1 k) In cases of suspected hydrocephalus where no ventricular dilatation could be demonstrated in the SEG, control examinations were performed for confirmation.

b) Results (compare Table 19)

In 36 of 50 subjects (72%), we were able to diagnose an enlarged ventricular system in the SEG.

2 a) Thirty of these 36 children exhibited macrocephalus, i. e., the circumference of the skull surpassed the 90th percentile level; 13 were progressive.

2 b) In 14 of the 30 macrocephali cases, signs of increased intracranial pressure further supported the suspicion of hydrocephalus.

2 c) In 15 of the 36 cases, the existence of hydrocephalus had been previously demonstrated in the PEG examination or at surgery. Although this was not taken into consideration in evaluating the group as a whole, we received reliable SEG confirmation of ventricular dilatation.

2 d) Six of 7 cases of extreme hydrocephalus with brain mantle thickness under 2 cm presented positive diaphane results.

2 e) We found inconspicuous cranial growth without the presence of macrocephalus in 2 cases.

2 f) Brain damage in early childhood or retardation of psychomotoric development was clinically found in 8 children exhibiting enlarged ventricles in the SEG. Such observations were also made by M. Jacobi and other authors.

In 9 children the expanse of the ventricular system determined by the SEG was found to be in the border range. Seven of these exhibited macrocephalus without progression, whereas 2 cases showed continuous progression. A single SEG examination was not sufficient in such cases, since progressive increase can be determined only by continuous examination.

Table 19. *Comparison of SEG results with clinical data. Abbreviations as follows: LV = lateral ventricles, VS = ventricular system, 3 V = third ventricle, BMT = brain mantle thickness, + = significant results, − = insignificant results, and ○ = data not available*

No.	SEG					Clinical data							
	Dilated 3 V	Dilated LV	Progressive expanse of VS	BMT 2 cm	Normal VS + VS in border area ++	Confirmed hydrocephalus	Noticeable cranial growth	Macrocephalus without progression	Progressive macrocephalus	Trans-illumination	Signs of brain pressure	Brain damage	Unremarkable
1	○	+	+	+	−	+	+	−	+	+	+	○	−
2	+	+	○	−	−	−	○	+	○	−	−	+	○
3	−	+	+	−	−	−	+	−	−	−	+	○	○
4	○	+	○	−	−	−	−	+	−	−	+	○	+
5	○	+	−	−	−	+	−	+	−	−	−	−	+
6	+	+	+	−	−	+	+	−	+	○	+	+	○
7	+	+	−	−	−	+	−	+	−	−	−	−	+
8	+	−	−	−	−	−	−	+	−	−	−	+	○
9	+	+	−	−	−	−	−	−	−	−	−	+	○
10	+	+	○	−	−	+	+	−	+	○	+	+	○
11	○	+	○	−	−	−	−	−	−	−	−	+	○
12	○	+	+	+	−	+	+	−	+	+	○	○	○
13	−	+	○	−	−	−	+	−	+	−	−	−	○
14	+	+	○	−	−	−	+	−	+	−	−	−	○
15	+	+	+	−	−	−	+	−	+	−	+	−	○
16	+	+	○	−	−	−	−	−	−	−	+	−	−
17	−	+	○	−	−	−	−	+	−	−	+	○	○
18	+	+	○	−	−	+	+	−	+	−	+	−	○
19	+	−	−	−	−	−	−	+	−	−	−	−	○
20	−	+	−	+	−	+	−	+	−	+	−	−	+
21	−	+	−	−	−	+	−	+	−	○	−	−	+
22	+	(+)	−	−	−	−	−	+	−	−	−	+	+
23	○	+	○	+	−	+	−	+	−	○	+	−	○
24	○	+	○	−	−	−	+	−	+	○	−	−	○
25	+	○	○	−	−	−	−	+	−	○	−	−	○
26	+	+	−	−	−	−	−	−	−	−	−	+	○
27	+	+	+	+	−	+	+	−	+	+	+	−	○
28	+	+	○	−	−	−	−	+	−	−	(+)	−	○
29	+	+	○	−	−	−	−	+	−	○	−	−	○
30	+	+	−	−	−	−	+	−	−	−	−	−	○
31	+	(+)	○	−	−	+	−	+	−	−	−	−	○
32	+	+	○	−	−	−	+	−	+	○	−	−	○
33	+	+	○	+	−	+	+	−	+	(+)	+	−	−
34	+	+	+	+	−	+	+	−	+	+	+	−	−
35	+	+	−	−	−	−	−	+	−	○	+	○	○
36	+	+	+	−	−	+	−	+	−	−	+	−	+
37	−	−	−	−	+	−	−	+	−	−	−	○	+
38	−	−	−	−	++	−	−	+	−	○	−	−	○
39	−	−	−	−	++	−	−	+	−	−	−	○	○
40	−	−	−	−	+	−	−	+	−	−	−	−	+
41	−	−	−	−	++	−	−	+	−	−	−	−	○
42	−	−	○	−	++	−	+	−	+	−	−	−	○
43	−	−	−	−	++	−	−	+	−	−	−	−	○
44	○	−	○	−	+	−	−	+	−	−	−	−	+
45	−	−	−	−	++	(+)	−	+	−	−	−	−	+
46	−	−	−	−	+	−	−	+	−	−	−	−	+
47	−	−	−	−	+	−	−	+	−	−	−	−	○
48	−	−	−	−	++	−	−	+	−	−	−	−	○
49	−	−	−	−	++	−	−	+	−	○	−	−	○
50	−	−	−	−	++	−	−	−	+	−	−	○	○

In 5 cases the SEG exhibited a normal ventricular system combined with stabilized macrocephalus.

The data in Table 19, as given above, is summarized in Table 20 and 21 in two different aspects.

In classifying the 36 children with normal SEG results and 9 children in the border range, we did not differentiate between individual results concerning clinical signs of an enlarged ventricular system, or as the case may be, of increased intracranial pressure.

In cases with progressive macrocephalus there was also evidence of conspicuous cranial growth. We considered these findings to be only signs (Table 21).

Table 20 demonstrates the following:

a) In all cases where more than one clinical sign was present, abnormal SEG results were found.

b) In cases where only one clinical sign was present, the SEG often demonstrated border range values.

Table 20. *Number of clinical signs compared to various SEG-results*

SEG results	No. of clinical signs indicating an enlarged ventricular system			
	4	3	2	1
Dilated ventricular system (36 cases)	14.2%	16.6%	33.2%	36.0%
Ventricular system in border range (9 cases)	0%	0%	0%	100%

Table 21. *Frequency of clinical signs compared with sonoencephalographic findings (%)*

Clinical signs	SEG findings		
	dilated ventricular system (36)	ventricular system in border range (9)	normal ventricular system (5)
Brain damage	22.2%	0%	0%
Signs of increased brain pressure	44.4%	0%	0%
Transillumination	16.6%	0%	0%
Macrocephalus with progression	36.0%	22.2%	0%
Macrocephalus without progression	46.5%	77.7%	100%
Noticeable cranial growth	41.6%	11.1%	0%
Confirmed hydrocephalus	41.6%	0%	0%

c) When the SEG examination revealed a ventricular system in the border range, no more than a clinical sign could be deduced.

Consequently, a good correlation is obtained between the number of clinical signs indicating hydrocephalus and abnormal SEG results.

How often did the presented clinical data confirm our SEG results of an enlarged ventricular system? Which clinical signs were most frequently present when SEG values showed the ventricular system to be in the border area, and which were most frequently present when normal values were exhibited (Table 21).

Table 21 demonstrates the following:

a) The most frequent clinical findings associated with abnormal SEG values were macrocephalus without progression.

b) Signs of increased cerebral pressure, noticeable increased cranial growth, and definite diagnosis of hydrocephalus are established at approximately the same time.

c) When the SEG resulted in a ventricular system in the border range, the most frequent clinical observation was macrocephalus.

With this method, a significant correlation between the type of clinical signs and the SEG results in hydrocephalus was demonstrated.

B. Comparison of SEG and PEG Measurements of the Third Ventricle

a) Determination of Comparative Values

Pneumoencephalograms from 60 children were included in the following series. In 15 PEGs the third ventricle was not sufficiently contrasted, in 4 cases neither SEG nor PEG values could be obtained, and in a further 4 cases the SEG examination was not successful.

In order to compare the remaining 37 cases, the diameter of the third ventricle (q) was measured on the PEG a-p film and compared to the corresponding diameter of the entire cranial diameter (Q). On the SEG film q was also measured, Q being determined by adding an age dependent constant K to the end echo. In order to compare the two procedures, divergence in the X-rays must be considered. This was accomplished by a simple calculation; namely, by establishing a relationship between the PEG width of the third ventricle and the PEG cranial diameter, and multiplying this by the SEG cranial diameter.

$$\frac{q_{PEG}}{Q_{PEG}} \times \frac{Q_{SEG}}{1} = X$$

The calculated values for X (Table 22) were compared to the SEG measurements of the width of the third ventricle. This was accomplished by placing the SEG values on the ordinate and the PEG values on the abscisse (Fig. 23).

Values indicating deviation of the two procedures were obtained in 5 cases. These are given in Table 22. In the coordinate system of Fig. 23, only the larger of the two measurements is given.

Table 22. *Sonoencephalographic and pneumoencephalographic values for third ventricular width (mm)*

No.	Name	SEG	PEG	No.	Name	SEG	PEG
1	B. T.	4	4.3	20	K. A.	5	6
2	B. A.	5	6.3	21	L. J.	4.5	4.8/3.6
3	E. U.	3.5	3.3	22	L. C.	5.5	5.3
4	E. H.	4	4	23	M. S.	4	4.1
5	F. H.	6	5.9	24	N. H.	8.5	8.6/7.5
6	F. E.	3	3.5	25	N. A.	4	5.6
7	G. J.	5	6.4/3.1	26	O. T.	3	3.9
8	G. M.	10	11.4/5.8	27	R. S.	4.5	5.5
9	G. M.	5.5	5.5	28	R. H.	2	2.6
10	G. N.	16	16	29	S. M.	4	4.7
11	G. G.	8	8.7	30	S. U.	6	7
12	G. C.	5	5.6	31	S. M.	5	5
13	H. S.	5.5	5.6	32	S. E.	5	5.3
14	H. S.	5.5	5.9	33	S. M.	5.5	6
15	H. S.	4	5.5	34	S. H.	18	18
16	H. C.	3	5	35	T. G.	4	3.7
17	H. R.	16	16.8	36	V. C.	6	6.4
18	H. U.	20	20	37	W. A.	7	6.8/4.3
19	K. S.	6	5.8				

b) Results

Thirty-one of 37 comparisons (83,8%) exhibited a correlation of ±1 mm. When a correlation of ±1.5 mm was considered, a further 4 patients are included (94.6%). The remaining 2 cases were found to be in the range of ±2 mm (100%). The correlation coefficient "r" was 0.93. The formula for the degree regression was $y = 0.01105 + 0.90290 \cdot x$. Normal values for the width of the third ventricle were found to be between 2.5 and 6 mm, depending upon the age of the patient (Fig. 10). Values over 7 mm were considered abnormal.

It can be seen from the distribution of the values given in Fig. 23 that as the third ventricle increases in size, the deviation in measurement was less. This observation can be easily explained, since the walls of the third ventricle become tense and smooth when under pressure. However, a statistically valid explanation cannot be given because of the small number of cases.

C. Comparison of Sonoencephalographic and Pneumoencephalographic Values of the Lateral Ventricle

In 33 of 60 cases (55%) included in this study, we obtained an exact measurement of the diameter of the lateral ventricles in the SEG and in the PEG.

In order to work with comparative values, we employed an index. This has the following advantages: 1. the relationships employed remain fairly constant throughout life, 2. observance of X-rays divergence is unnecessary, and 3. this method has proven more useful in follow-up studies, since the index remains almost constant during physiological growth of the skull and ventricular system.

1. Calculation of the SEG Lateral Ventricular Index (LVI)

First, we determined the diameter of both lateral ventricles (d) from the SEG film by measuring the distance between the echoes originating from the outer walls of the lateral ventricles (LV_1, LV_2). Next, the cranial diameter (D) was determined by adding an age dependent constant K for the thickness of the osseous cranium (Fig. 7) to the value of the end echo (EE), which originates from the far side inner table. The lateral ventricular index was calculated from the relationship between the width of the lateral ventricles and the entire cranial diameter.

$$I_{SEG} = \frac{(\text{distance } LV_1 \text{ to } LV_2)}{(\text{distance IE to EE}) + K} = \frac{d}{D}$$

2. Evaluation of PEGs (Fig. 37)

All measurements were made from pneumoencephalographic a-p films of examinations performed with the patient in the supine position. An index comparable to the sonoencephalographic LVI was calculated by measuring the width of the lateral ventricles and the corresponding cranial diameter.

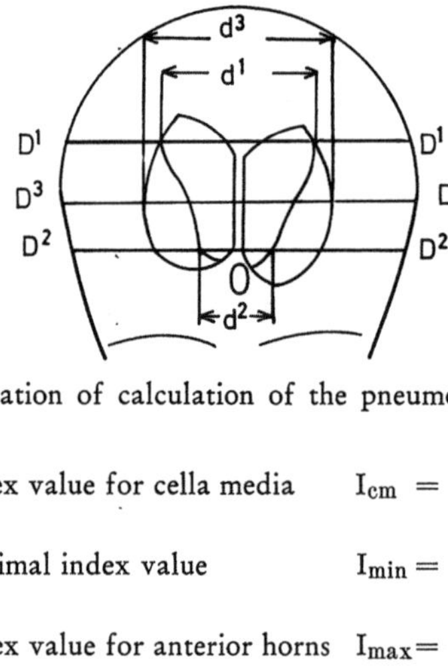

Fig. 37. Schematic representation of calculation of the pneumoencephalographic lateral ventricular index.

Index value for cella media $I_{cm} = \frac{d_1}{D_1}$

Minimal index value $I_{min} = \frac{d_2}{D_2}$

Index value for anterior horns $I_{max} = \frac{d_3}{D_3}$

A pneumoencephalographic lateral ventricular index was measured from the following three horizontal planes:

1. index value of the cella media (I_{cm}),
2. minimal index value (I_{min}), and
3. index value of the anterior horns (I_{max}).

I_{cm} was measured, because at this position the corresponding walls of the lateral ventricles are farthest apart.

I_{min} was measured from the smallest point of the cella media. In determining values from this plane, we employed an SEG-principle; namely, that it is only possible to represent both outer walls of the lateral ventricles simultaneously when the ultrasonic waves are reflected perpendicularly from each structure.

Measurements from this position could not always be determined, since the angle of inclination of the lateral ventricular outer walls gradually changes toward the ventricular floor. Nevertheless, we established an index from this plane in order to have some orientation concerning lowermost border values for comparison purposes. This could be thought of as the lowest possible beam plane.

I_{max} was measured from the widest point of the a-p film, which was normally in the anterior horn area. This represented a border value also for orientation purposes, since the normal reference plane in the SEG examination is the cella media.

3. Comparison of PEG and SEG Lateral Ventricular Index

The calculated SEG and PEG values are compared in Table 23. We considered SEG values significant when the sonoencephalographic index (I_{SEG}) was found to be the same as or between I_{max} and I_{min}.

Table 23. *Sonoencephalographic and pneumoencephalographic index values for lateral ventricular width. Abbreviations:* I_{max} *= maximal PEG index value,* I_{cm} *= PEG index measured at the cella media,* I_{min} *= minimal PEG index value,* I_{SEG} *= sonoencephalographic index*

	Name	Age	I_{max}	I_{cm}	I_{min}	I_{SEG}
1	S. A.	10 y.	0.26	0.20	0.10	0.26
2	S. M.	13 y.	0.25	0.21	0.12	0.25
3	N. H.	3 y.	0.23	0.23	0.15	0.40
4	E. E.	5 y.	0.27	0.24	0.12	0.23
5	J. A.	10 y.	0.27	0.24	0.12	0.27
6	S. U.	2 y.	0.27	0.25	0.17	0.24
7	A. S.	1 y.	0.37	0.27	—	0.30
8	L. C.	8 m.	0.29	0.28	0.14	0.21
9	E. U.	4 y.	0.32	0.28	0.12	0.25
10	O. T.	7 m.	0.28	0.28	0.15	0.28
11	R. S.	7 m.	0.33	0.28	0.18	0.28
12	P. P.	3 m.	0.31	0.28	0.16	0.31
13	H. S.	1 y.	0.35	0.29	0.16	0.24
14	W. A.	5 y.	0.32	0.29	0.18	0.28
15	R. H.	4 m.	0.30	0.30	0.19	0.29
16	S. E.	5 y.	0.32	0.30	0.18	0.30
17	S. M.	6 m.	0.34	0.31	0.22	0.25
18	L. M.	9 m.	0.31	0.31	0.18	0.28
19	M. S.	1 y.	0.34	0.31	0.16	0.32
20	H. S.	8 m.	0.42	0.32	0.16	0.27
21	M. S.	5 m.	0.32	0.32	0.16	0.29
22	N. A.	2 m.	0.38	0.32	0.10	0.31
23	W. M.	4 m.	0.46	0.32	—	0.42
24	S. A.	7 y.	0.33	0.32	0.14	0.26
25	H. C.	2 y.	0.38	0.33	0.20	0.32
26	G. C.	3 y.	0.37	0.35	0.16	0.32
27	V. C.	1 y.	0.40	0.38	0.17	0.30
28	G. J.	10 m.	0.55	0.38	—	0.46
29	E. D.	9 m.	0.45	0.39	—	0.39
30	S. M.	10 y.	0.51	0.51	0.28	0.42
31	H. J.	9 y.	0.52	0.52	0.52	0.52
32	G. G.	6 y.	0.54	0.54	0.54	0.55
33	H. R.	1 y.	0.55	0.55	0.55	0.57

In 4 cases we were able to determine I_{max} and I_{cm} but not I_{min}. In such cases we considered a significant correlation to be present when I_{SEG} was between the pneumoencephalographic I_{max} and I_{cm} or exhibited a value close to I_{cm}.

The results of the measurements presented in Table 23 are summarized in Fig. 38. In employing these values, we examined the correlation between SEG and PEG measurements of the lateral ventricles. We recorded on the ordinate in each individual case the area between I_{max} and I_{min} as vertical lines, each containing also the value for I_{cm} and I_{SEG}. In 30 of 33 cases (91%) we could demonstrate a valid correlation between the two examination procedures (Fig. 38). In 2 of 3 remaining

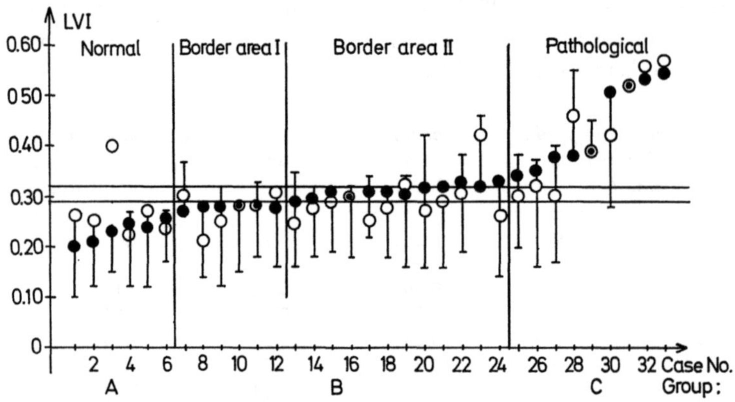

Fig. 38. Graphical demonstration of the tabulated values for I_{max} and I_{min} in 33 cases from Table 23 (I_{min} and I_{max} are connected by vertical lines). I_{SEG} and I_{cm} are classified according to SCHIERSMANN: A = normal ventricular system; B = border area I and II; C = pathologically dilated ventricular system; ○ = I_{SEG}; ● = I_{cm}

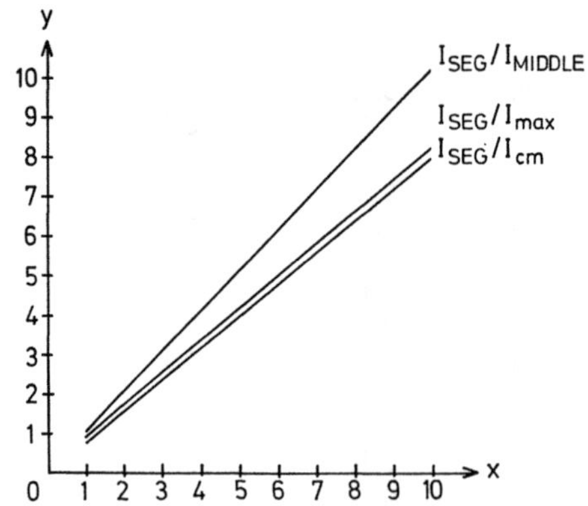

Fig. 39. Regression curve for the relationships between I_{SEG} and I_{PEG} (I_{max}, I_{cm}, and $I_{middle} = \frac{I_{max}+I_{min}}{2}$). The appropriate formulas are as follows:

I_{SEG}/I_{max} $\quad y=0.0984+0.8143\,x_1$

I_{SEG}/I_{cm} $\quad y=0.0669+0.7991\,x_2$

$I_{SEG}\ \frac{I_{max}+I_{min}}{2}$ $\quad y=0.0413+1.0421\,x_3$

cases (No. 32 and 33), which did not offer this criteria, extreme hydrocephalus was present. Furthermore, in these cases I_{SEG} was only slightly larger than I_{max} (0.57 and 0.55, and 0.55 and 0.54 respectively). In the third patient (No. 3), the comparison with air studies revealed that the trigonum collaterale was situated in an extreme anterior position; consequently, examination from the reference line produced the trigonum collaterale instead of the cella media.

Calculation of the coefficient of correlation for the various relationships I_{SEG} to I_{PEG} yielded the following values:

$$I_{SEG}/I_{max} \quad \text{"r"} = 0.82$$
$$I_{SEG}/I_{cm} \quad \text{"r"} = 0.83$$
$$I_{SEG}/\frac{I_{max}+I_{min}}{2} \quad \text{"r"} = 0.95$$

In can be observed that the closest relationship exists between I_{SEG} and the arithmetical average from $I_{max}+I_{min}$ (Fig. 21). Fig. 39 reveals the rate of regression for the three relationships I_{SEG} to I_{PEG}.

D. Comparison of the Roentgenological and Sonoencephalographical Lateral Ventricular Index

The question concerning the diagnostic value of indices obtained from the cella media area is of cardinal importance when only values from this area are available to the examiner. Consequently, we examined the value of unidimensional ultrasonic representation of the lateral ventricles. Assessment of the cerebral ventricles was based on the results of the combined SEG-PEG examinations described above (see Fig. 38).

Employment of lateral ventricular indices has been known in roentgenology since its introduction by SCHIERSMANN. He has established the following three categories for index results: normal, borderline and abnormal. In Fig. 38 we proceeded in a similar fashion to categorize our results. Ascending values for I_{cm} have been numbered from 1 to 33 and grouped into categories A, B and C.

Group A comprises values up to 0.25 (corresponding SCHIERSMANN value = 4.0) which SCHIERSMANN considers normal.

Group C values over 0.33 (corresponding to 3.0) are viewed as absolutely abnormal.

Group B is composed of cases where it is uncertain whether the width of the lateral ventricles may be considered normal or abnormal, or whether further parameters are necessary to establish a diagnosis. This group exhibited index values for I_{cm} between 0.25 and 0.32 (analogous to 3.0 to 4.0). SCHIERSMANN divided these values into the following two groups: First, those exhibiting index values between 0.25 and 0.285 (=4.0 to 3.5). These ventricular values were described as "bulky but still within the normal range." Secondly, those values between 0.285 and 0.33 were interpreted by SCHIERSMANN to be a sign of "mild dilatation of the lateral ventricles that can be considered abnormal in most cases."

At this time we compared the SEG lateral ventricular indices to those obtained by the PEG. The following conclusions could be made.

In 8 cases I_{SEG} was found to be in the normal range and I_{cm} in the border range. Twenty-three cases exhibited I_{cm} values in the uppermost border area and I_{SEG} values in the normal range. Small differences between I_{SEG} and I_{cm} cannot be avoided. In SEG representation of the lateral ventricles, the examination is carried out from a uniform position on the external skull and, consequently, it is understandable that exact correlation of the SEG reference plane and the roentgenological plane would only be due to chance. Significant differences that could lead to complete misinterpretation are not expected and, as shown in Fig. 38, were not present in our series.

Examination Results

The SEG results correlate in general with the classification proposed by SCHIERSMANN.

A) Normal

B) Border range

C) Abnormal

The radiologist has the advantage of additional criteria in evaluation of the lateral ventricles in their true perspective, since he possesses access to the X-ray film depicting the typical butterfly figure, curvature of the external corners, and the abundance of contrast media in the most anterior portion of the anterior horns. On the other hand, the SEG examiner has only index values at his disposal in his evaluation of the lateral ventricles. Further parameters which can aid in his evaluation are the expanse of the third ventricle and of the temporal horns.

In total assessment of roentgenological a-p films of the lateral ventricles, it can be seen that in the present material the evaluation of "bulky" or "slightly enlarged lateral ventricles" was given starting at $I_{cm} = 0.28$. Considering all aspects, case 24 with $I_{cm} = 0.32$ can be evaluated as normal. MOSTAFAWY and WINTER reported normal values in children with LVI up to 0.32.

Our examination confirms the merit of the lateral ventricular index. SJÖGREN reports an index value of 0.30 which should not be surpassed in normal cases. However, this value does not appear to be adequate as a border between normal and abnormal values in the examination under consideration. In the SEG examination, as well as in radiology, border range values must be standardized, whereby index values from 0.29 to 0.32 can be considered as "bulky to slightly dilated" for clinical purposes. When considering whether the lateral ventricles are normally or abnormally enlarged, one must take other parameters into consideration (BMI, third ventricle, and head circumference).

E. The Value of SEG Follow-up Studies in Evaluation of Hydrocephalus

The value of the SEG in follow-up studies has often been confirmed and emphasized (JEPPSON, BRÜCKNER, etc.). In the diagnosis of hydrocephalus, this possibility of measuring the ventricular system in vivo within the shortest possible time period is of great value, especially when it is a question of progression. Ultrasonic representation of the width of the cerebral ventricles is, in fact, the only method in which the width of these structures can be continuously checked after a spinal fluid by-pass operation.

Illustrative Cases

The purpose of the following series of cases is to establish the merit of SEG follow-up examinations in detecting increases and decreases in ventricular width.

Case No. 3

V. A., born July, 21, 1968, File No. 4175/68. This $2^1/_2$ week premature infant exhibited macrocephalus at birth (head circumference = 30.5 cm / −4.5 cm). Cranial growth was progressive and approached the normal curve. On Sept. 5, diaphany of the cranial vault showed transillumination, and the PEG on Dec. 9 exhibited hydrocephalus and porencephaly. The SEG follow-up films are presented in Fig. 40.

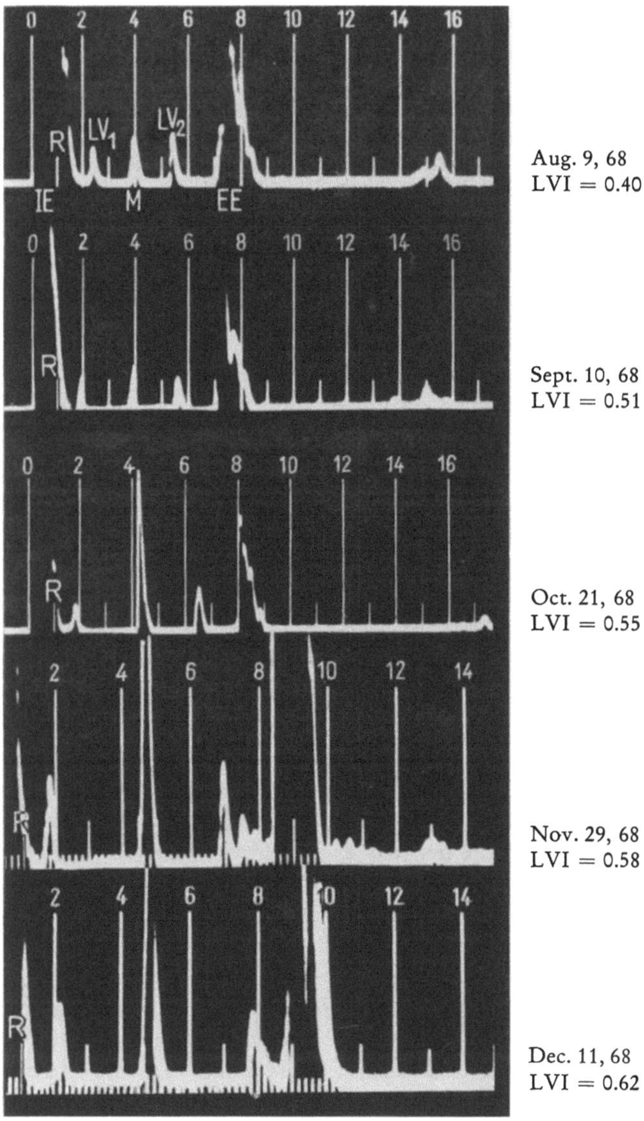

Fig. 40. SEG follow-up study in a child with progressive hydrocephalus. Lateral ventricular index values increase from 0.40 to 0.62 within 4 months

Case No. 4

M. A., born Nov. 23, 1963, File No. 7506/68. This four-and-one-half year old male was born with a cranial circumference of 45 cm, 10 cm above the average. Since the cranial circumference increased at a noticeable rate, a surgical by-pass of the spinal fluid (Spitz-Holter valve) was performed at 7 weeks of age. The operation was successful, and further development was satisfactory. SEG follow-up examinations were undertaken at $4^1/_2$ years of age and continued for 2 months. The patient exhibited an extremely enlarged ventricular system (LVI = 0.68); however, no significant progression was evident. The child displays above average capabilities.

In the following two cases we examined whether reaction of the brain parenchyma to pressure variations is observable within a few hours.

Case No. 5

U. S., born April 24, 1968, File No. 2961/69. This child was born with congenital hydrocephalus. A ventriculographic examination carried out 3 weeks later showed extreme hydrocephalus. On May 21, 1969, a Spitz-Holter valve was introduced. Following the operation, the cranial bones began overlapping. Four months later the valve was removed because of sepsis. Following this, the cranial circumference increased rapidly in spite of the fact that direct ventricular punctures for pressure alleviation were undertaken almost daily.

In summary, the clinical course in this case took the following form: 24 days to pressure alleviation, 4 months later removal of valve followed by pressure increase, followed by periodic pressure alleviation via direct ventricular puncture. Twenty-six days following removal of the valve, we carried out daily SEG examinations in which we concentrated on presentation of the brain mantle thickness from 4 marked reference points. This extended over a 5-day period. On the first day, SEG examination was performed prior to puncture, and on the following days, 2, 4, 6, and 10 hours after puncture. By measuring brain mantle thickness within such a short time after puncture, we could find no reaction of the brain parenchyme to pressure alleviation.

Case No. 6

A. L., born Feb. 23, 1968, File No. 3060/69. This child exhibited congenital hydrocephalus. A shunt operation was performed on Sep. 11, 1969, at the age of $6^1/_2$ months. The valve remained only 12 days, after which time sepsis necessitated removal. Cranial circumference increased rapidly post-operative.

In this case the pressure increase remained for a longer period and the pressure alleviation pursued more rapidly (12 days). During the 5-day SEG control series, punctures were performed only on the first and last days. The sonic beaming procedure was performed on the first day shortly before puncture and on the fifth day 10 hours thereafter.

Remarkable changes in brain tissue could not be demonstrated in either of the above cases. Variations in the brain mantle thickness were registered from the probe side. However, since these variations exhibited the exact opposite reaction as would be expected on the basis of alterations in pressure relationships, and, since they were in contradiction to the unchanged value obtained in the region near the probe, one cannot place much value in these results. These values can best be explained by the fact that, although the examinations were carried out from the same reference point, a somewhat different probe-scalp angle was probably used; thereby, different sections of the irregular brain mantle were dealt with.

In the following case, a significant reaction of the brain parenchyma to pressure increases and decreases over a period of several days can be demonstrated.

Case No. 7

E. J., born April 13, 1969, File No. 2509/69. This patient, a one-week old girl, was admitted due to complications arising from a compound breech presentation, with prolapse of an arm. 24 hours post-partum the child was screaming loudly and had clonic convulsions. On examination, the fontanelles were slightly distended, and hypertension was discovered. The diagnosis of intracranial hematoma arising from birth trauma was established. The bleeding impaired the absorption of liquor in the periphery, the pressure increased and the cranial circumference expanded. With the first spinal punctures undertaken for pressure alleviation, the liquor was dark red. With each subsequent puncture the color of the liquor became lighter, until only xanthochromic coloration was observed. Cranial circumference ceased to expand and the fontanelles were no longer distended. Further punctures were unnecessary. The increasing expanse in the lateral ventricles and their subsequent decrease were followed in the SEG (Fig. 41 a and 41 b).

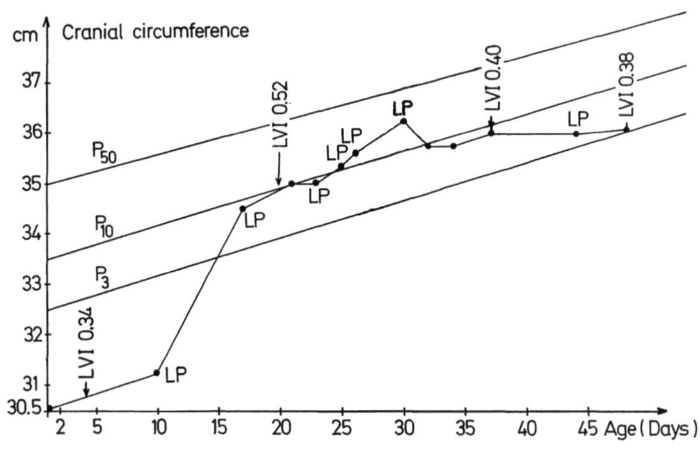

Fig. 41 a. SEG findings as compared to cranial circumference. Increase and decrease in liquor pressure after birth-traumatic intracranial hemorrhage can be followed (Case No. 7, born on April 13, 1969). Abbreviations: LVI = Lateral ventricle index; LP = Lumbal puncture; P = percentile

Case No. 8

Alexander K., 12 months old, File No. 5610/69, was treated on an outpatient basis between April 20 and Aug. 1, 1968, for repeated infections. During the last examination, it was noticed that cranial circumference had increased to 49 cm—about 1.2 cm above the 90th percentile. The fontanelles and the cranial sutures were clearly open. During the present examination, it was noticed that this one-year old child demonstrated poor posture and that the claviculae were absent on palpation. These findings led to further roentgenologic studies, at which time the diagnosis of pelvicocleidocranialis dysostosis was established. During hospitalization (because of suspected hydrocephalus), the cranial circumference increased to 53 cm—2 cm above the 90th percentile. Examination of internal systems was negative.

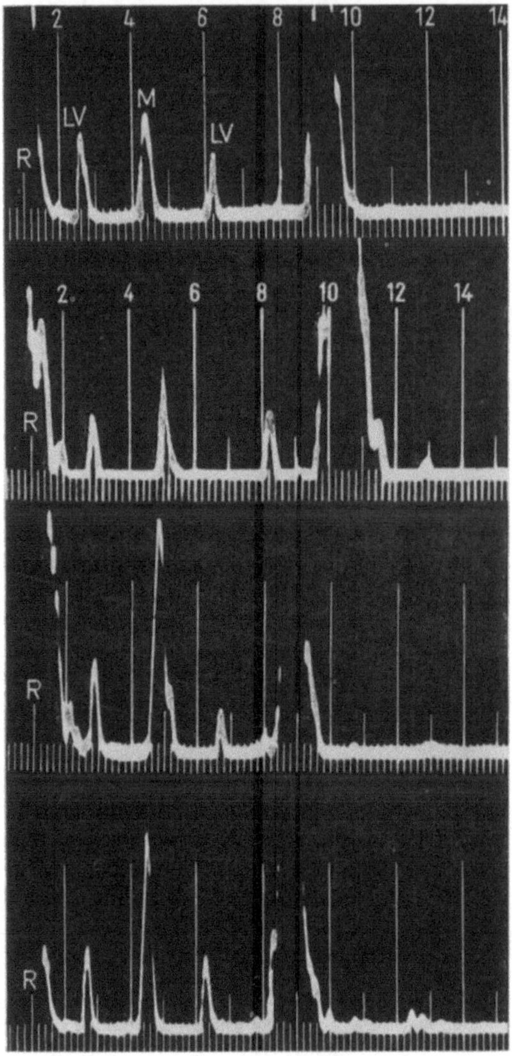

LVI = 0.34

LVI = 0.52

LVI = 0.40

LVI = 0.38

Fig. 41 b. SEG follow-up study demonstrates the decreasing width of the lateral ventricles with alleviation of liquor pressure (Case No. 7)

Neurological status: Cranial nerve as well as sensory examination was negative. Seizures were denied and no alteration in reflex activity or any symptoms of basilar impression were observed.

EEG: Basal activity corresponding to patient age; no focal abnormalities.

SEG: Follow-up studies demonstrated an increase in the lateral ventricular index from 0.30 to 0.37 which corresponds to PEG values (Fig. 42).

Diagnosis: Pelvicocleidocranial dysostosis and internal hydrocephalus.

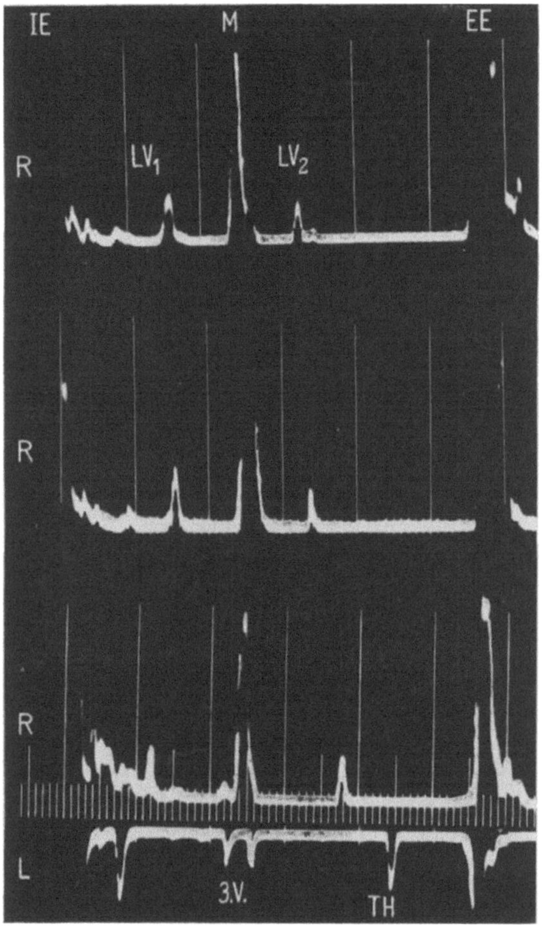

Fig. 42. Sonoencephalographic follow-up studies of a boy with pelvicocleidocranial dystosis and hydrocephalus (Case No. 8). The lateral ventricular index (LVI) increased from 0.30 to 0.37 within 15 months. The brain mantle index (BMI), calculated from the temporal horn outer wall (TH) was 2.8. Abbreviations: IE = initial echo, M = midline echo, EE = end echo, 3.V. = third ventricle, and LV = lateral ventricle outer wall

XIII. Sources of Error and Particulars

Prior to the interpretation of each SEG examination, the examiner must be well orientated concerning possible sources of error; namely, objective, technical and subjective conditions determined by the examiner. The method has its definite limitations, and one should not succumb to the tendency of loosely applying his own interpretations.

Unavoidable errors arising from laws of physics have their origin in the fact that the sonic reflections present all acoustical interfaces in an identical manner on the oscilloscope screen, without depicting morphology of the structures. Since sonic reflections cannot easily be manipulated, the possible subjective sources of error decrease as the examiner gathers experience. Therefore, much experience on the part of the examiner is imperative, in order to evaluate the individual reflections correctly. Table 24 summarizes the structures and anomalies which, according to our experiences, represent the most frequent sources of error.

Table 24. *Summary of possible sources of error. Structures and anomalies that can lead to misinterpretation and confusion of midline echoes, lateral ventricular index, brain mantle index and third ventricular echoes*

Cerebral falx *Septum pellucidum*	a) unilateral enlargement of cranium b) walls of the third ventricle, when only one wall can be demonstrated in scanning c) cranial asymmetry d) walls of the cavum septi pellucidi e) lateral position of hydrocephalics during examination
Lateral ventricles *Temporal horns*	a) unusual high positions of the temporal horns b) insular cyst in the lateral fissure c) cysts d) subdural hygroma
Third ventricle	a) septum pellucidum cavity b) cysts in the region of the third ventricle

a
b

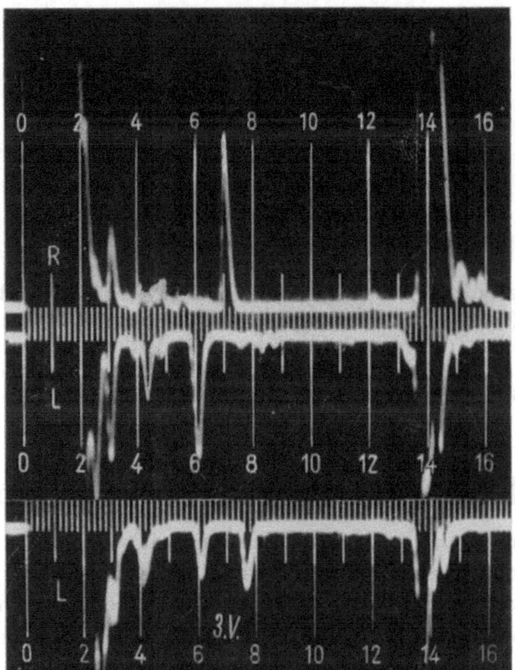

Fig. 43. Unauthentic midline echo shifts associated with third ventricular dilatation. The unauthentic midline shift demonstrated in the upper film represents the midline echo, as detected from the right side (a), and one wall of the third ventricle, as detected from the left side (b). Both walls of the third ventricle are demonstrated in the lower film (3.V.)

A. Erroneous Measurement in Determining the Midline Echo

The following can lead to erroneous measurement:

a) Unilateral extracranial soft tissue swelling of different etiology, e. g., scalp hematomas or phlegmonas can cause apparent midline displacement in bitemporal beaming, which must be considered in evaluation of the midline echo.

b) A dilated third ventricle can lead to apparent displacement in the midline echo, since only one of the lateral walls of the third ventricle can be taken for the midline echo in each bitemporal examination. Similarly, representation of one wall of the third ventricle and the midline echo can produce a film with delusive midline shift (Fig. 43).

c) Cranial asymmetry.

d) Walls of the septum pellucidum cavity.

e) Performing the SEG examination with the hydrocephalic child lying on his side. The weight of the liquor in the hydrocephalic child in this position causes false representation. In connection with this SJÖGREN refers to the importance of the supine position.

B. Sources of Error in Measuring the Width of the Third Ventricle

Although the competent examiner has no difficulty representing the characteristic double echo originating from the walls of the third ventricle, the following factors can lead to misinterpretation of SEG measurements:

a) Cysts in the cavum vergae.

b) Cysts of the septum pellucidum.

c) Misinterpretation in cases of dilated third ventricles. This occurs by confusing the midline echo with reflections from an outer wall of the lateral ventricle or misinterpreting the reflections from one wall of the third ventricle and one wall of the lateral ventricle, both of which can be taken to present the characteristic double echo. However, this can be corrected by presenting both outer walls of the lateral ventricles on the oscilloscope screen in order to provide structural orientation.

C. Sources of Error in Determining the Lateral Ventricular and Brain Mantle Index

The anatomical form of the lateral ventricles exhibits distinct individual differences. Moreover, only portions of the outer walls of the lateral ventricles are parallel to the cranial bones, as is the case in the area of the cella media and the inferior horns. Only in the latter positions can SEG measurement be obtained without difficulty.

When examining the area of the cella media, only a small portion of the lateral ventricles can be measured; however, this portion is decisive, since:

a) the anterior horns and the cella media represent the least amount of individual deviation,

b) in ventricular dilation the anterior horns and the cella media are affected more strongly and at an earlier stage than the temporal horns (Fig. 44), and

c) in the abnormal case the lateral ventricles dilate the most and at a more constant rate than the other portions of the ventricular system.

SEG representation of the outer walls of the temporal horns is of great significance. SCHIEFER and KAZNER reported that the inferior horns expand in a definitive relationship to the cella media, so that it is possible to assess dilation of the entire ventricular system in accordance with temporal horn dilation. However, it has been our experience that this method of ventricular representation in pediatrics poses several problems. Above all, the numerous additional reflections, such as lateral and insular echoes in the area of the inferior horns, often complicate clear delineation of the desired structures. Therefore, we prefer measuring the lateral ventricular index

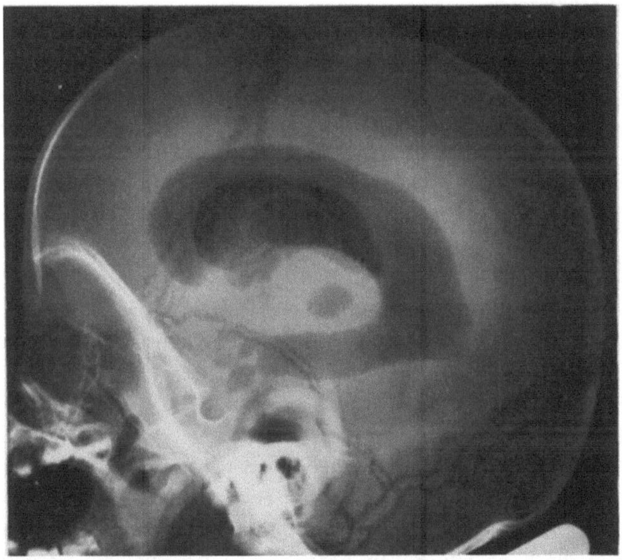

Fig. 44. A lateral pneumoencephalogram film demonstrating lateral ventricles which are more strongly affected in the area of the anterior horn and cella media than in the area of the temporal horns. These finding agrees with our general observations

which can be more easily determined during childhood. We have presented the reliability of this procedure in evaluating the width of the ventricular system (Ch. XII).

In the area of the cella media, different values for ventricular width can be obtained when the examination is carried out from different reference points. Since this represents a possible source of error, especially in follow-up examinations, we usually attempt to carry out the examination of the lateral ventricles in each child from a single reference point. Should the outer walls of the lateral ventricles be presented from a different position, we note it on the back side of the SEG film. This has the advantage of enabling additional examinations to be performed from the same position even if the procedure is carried out by different examiners.

Part Three: The Combined EEG and SEG

XIV. The Combined Electroencephalographic and Sonoencephalographic Examination

A. Introduction

EEG alterations in intracranial space-occupying lesions are manifold with variations appearing as local or diffuse changes. Localized symptoms are the direct result of neoplastic tissue in the cerebral cortex; those referred to as diffuse symptoms are the sequelae of intracranial tissue displacement, increased pressure on the brain, etc.

During childhood, electrical abnormalities in addition to those described above, e. g., *intermittent delta activity* and *confusing delta foci,* which are usually localized in the posterior region of the brain, often complicate localization and lateralization of a lesion.

Diversified opinions exist as to the diagnostic effectiveness of the EEG in intracranial space-occupying lesions during childhood. While BOLDREY et al. were disenchanted with EEG findings in their series of childhood tumors, TÖNNIS et al. interpreted their findings in tumors of the hemispheres to be reliable criteria.

When only electroencephalographic results are available, even when a lateralized and localized focus can be demonstrated, the following differential diagnostic possibilities remain:

a) unilateral space-occupying lesion,
b) localized atrophical changes,
c) localized symptom of a deep-seated lesion,
d) unilateral defect in cerebral circulation
(various congenital vascular defects, etc.).

It is obvious that the clinician may be confronted with further diagnostic difficulties, such as determining from which side to perform angiography.

Since electrical abnormalities are usually manifested in the form of focal EEG alterations (which present interpretation difficulties, particularly in children) further examinations are required in order to establish a definite diagnosis.

Before employing potentially dangerous contrast procedures, such as angiography, pneumoencephalography, or scintiscanning, sonoencephalography should be performed. When sonoencephalography alone is undertaken, it cannot be determined whether lateral tissue displacement occurs as the result of

a) an atrophical lesion in the hemisphere towards the midline shift, or
b) a space occupying lesion in the opposite hemisphere.

The EEG-SEG can be considered as complementary examinations, since it is often the case that findings in one examination can often be more correctly interpreted when results of the other examination are known. This is especially true when defining focal EEG changes and SEG midline shifts. The two procedures can also be performed in one sitting, representing a minimum of risk to the patient.

It is the purpose of this chapter to access the merit of the combined EEG-SEG examination.

EEG registration was performed with a 12-channel direct recorder by Schwarzer (recording speed of 30 m/sec, calibrated height of 7 mm or 50 mv, time constant usually 0.3 with a frequence opening of 30). We utilized bipolar longitudinal and transverse leads; and in the majority of cases, additional unipolar leads were recorded, employing the ear on the same side as the indifferent electrode. Recording time was usually 20 min. The majority of recordings was performed with the patient supine, and the remainder either with the patient in a half-sitting position with the head propped or fully sitting. Hyperventilation and photostimulation were employed as means of provocation.

Sonoencephalographic examinations were performed with the apparatus described on page 14.

B. Sonoencephalographic Examination Procedure

Sonoencephalography offers various examination possibilities. This is demonstrated in the following SEG parameters which were routinely determined in each patient:

a) position of diencephalic midline structures,
b) lateral ventricular width, and
c) third ventricular width.

A prerequisite was that at least two pictures be obtained in each case with clear delineation of reflections.

1. Position of Diencephalic Midline

Before determining the midline echo, cranial diameter was measured with a set of callipers. Half of this value was considered the theoretical brain midline (see p. 15). A pointer was fixed on the oscilloscope scale at this point, as well as at the position representing the diameter of the skull. In this manner, we could determine the expected position of the midline echo in each patient before examination.

In order to measure the midline echo, the probe was placed approximately 1.5 cm above the ear. Examination was performed from each side of the skull with photographic documentation of each midline echo (Fig. 8). In exceptional cases with cranial bone deformities, it was necessary to move the probe slightly anterior, posterior, or possibly, more to the top of the temporal bone.

Midline shifts of 2 mm were considered suspicious when the skull was symmetrical and corresponding EEG abnormalities were absent. Identical midline displacement was interpreted to be definitely abnormal when altered EEG patterns and concording clinical signs were present.

2. Determination of Lateral Ventricular Expanse

In order to locate reflections originating from the outer walls of the lateral ventricles, the probe was placed 4—5 cm above the external auditory meatus, i. e., on the upper border of the squamous portion of the temporal bone. By slightly rocking and gently moving the transducer's head, it is possible to synchronously demonstrate reflections from both outer walls of the lateral ventricles. In a few cases this examination technique enabled us to further demonstrate the temporal horn on the probe-opposite side. The usual procedure was to represent the midline echo along with the lateral ventricles and photographically record them on the upper half of the SEG film (Fig. 13). When ventricular asymmetry was suspected, repeated follow-up examinations were performed in order to exlude faulty projection of the examining beam.

Lateral ventricular values were expressed as indices resulting from the following calculation:

$$LVI = \frac{\text{expanse } LV_1 \text{ to } LV_2}{EE+K} = \frac{d}{D}$$

where d = distance between lateral ventricular echoes,
D = expanse between initial echo (IE) and end echo (EE), plus an age dependent constant (K) representing the thickness of the osseous cranium.
Distances on the SEG film are expressed in millimeters (Fig. 13).

3. Measuring Third Ventricular Width

The sonic probe was placed in the usual manner on the lower portion of the temple, slightly above and in front of the ear. After demonstrating the typical M-formed echo from both sides of the skull, it was registered in the lower portion of the SEG film (Fig. 13).

A *sonoventriculogram* was performed in the above manner, enabling evaluation of the ventricular system in each case. Lateral ventricular indices above 0.32 were considered significant, according to examinations reported by MOSTAFAWY et al. Third ventricular values over 7 mm were also interpreted as abnormal in concordance with the International Symposium on Echoencephalography, April 11, 1967, in Erlangen, Germany.

C. Subject Material

The following combined EEG-SEG studies include 100 patients varying in age from early infancy to 16 years, who were referred to our department during a two-year span beginning in February, 1968. An intracranial space-occupying lesion was suspected in each case. All patients presented significant indications such as headache, vomiting and seizures of unknown etiology. However, the classical symptom trias of brain tumor (headache, vomiting and papilledema) was not present in every case. Further neuroradiological contrast examinations were performed only when either of the examinations resulted in abnormal findings.

Table 25 presents the final diagnosis for the 100 subjects involved in this study.

Table 25. *Final diagnosis of 100 patients initially suspected of having an intracranial space-occupying lesion*

Final diagnosis	No. of cases
Supratentorial lesion	12
Infratentorial lesion	8
Cerebral atrophy	3
Various neurological conditions	77
Total	100

Confirmation of an intracranial space-occupying lesion was possible in 20 cases (20%), whereby the diagnosis was verified at surgery in 11 cases, and at autopsy in 6 cases. The anatomical location and microscopical findings in these 20 cases are presented in Table 26. Unilateral cerebral atrophy was discovered in 3 patients. The

Table 26. *Microscopical findings and anatomical location of the supra- and infratentorial brain tumors*

Supratentorial in location		Infratentorial in location	
Histology of lesion	Exact location	Histology of lesion	Exact location
Glioma	tectum opticum	—	pons
Sympaticoblastoma	generalized metastases	—	pons
		Glioblastoma	pons
Meningioma	temporal lobe	Astrocytoma	pons
Ependymoma	parieto-temporal	—	pons
Astrocytoma	temporal lobe	Spongioblastoma	cerebellar vermis
Astrocytoma	frontal lobe		
Oligodendroglioma	left hemisphere	Medulloblastoma	cerebellum
—	in third ventricle	Ependymoma	cerebellum
Ependymoma	basal ganglia		
Abscess	precentral		
—	midbrain		
Craniopharyngioma	suprasellular		
Total	12	Total	8

remaining 77 patients were found to have other neurological disturbances, such as epilepsy, hydrocephalus or meningoencephalitis.

D. EEG Results

The EEG revealed foci of slow wave activity in 7 of 12 patients (58.3%) with a supratentorial space-occupying lesion (Table 27). These 7 comprised 35% of all patients with focal changes observed in this series. A supratentorial mass was subsequently discovered in 3 of the 11 subjects (27.2%) exhibiting diffuse and dysrhythmic alterations. A similar diagnosis was established in 2 of the 69 patients (2.9%) exhibiting normal EEGs.

In the 8 subjects possessing an infratentorial tumor, no focal EEG abnormalities were recorded, although 6 patients (75%) exhibited diffuse electrical alteration. Normal EEG activity was discovered in 2 patients (25%) in this group.

Table 27. *EEG findings in 100 patients suspected of having an intracranial space-occupying lesion*

EEG findings	No. of cases	Supra-tentorial lesion	Infra-tentorial lesion	Atrophy	Various neurological disorders
Focal changes	20	7	0	3	10
Diffuse changes	11	3	6	0	2
Normal	69	2	2	0	65
Total	100	12	8	3	77

Unilateral cerebral atrophy was responsible for focal EEG abnormalities in 3 cases.

The reported data illustrate the extent to which a diagnosis can be established on the basis of EEG abnormalities alone. In the initial stage, supratentorial expanding lesions in children produce localized changes in the EEG. However, at a later stage, diffuse slowing and dysrhythmia predominate, so that exact localization and lateralization can no longer be determined from the EEG examination alone.

E. SEG Results

Results of sonoencephalographic examination of 100 patients with a suspected intracranial space-occupying lesion are summarized in Table 28. SEG results were interpreted as normal when the midline echo shift was under 2 mm, third ventricular width under 7 mm and the lateral ventricular index smaller than 0.31.

Table 28. *SEG results of 100 patients suspected of possessing an intracranial space-occupying lesion*

SEG findings		Total No. of cases (100)	Supra-tentorial (12 cases)	Infra-tentorial (8 cases)	Atrophy (3 cases)
Midline echo shift	> 2 mm	15	8	2	2
	= 2 mm	2	2	—	—
	< 2 mm	83	2	6	1
Lateral ventricles	dilated	20	9	8	—
	asymmetrical	5	—	—	1
	normal	72	2	—	2
	not measured	3	1	—	—
Third ventricle	dilated	18	6	8	—
	normal	75	3	—	—
	not measured	7	3	—	—

Diencephalic midline displacement of 2 mm with concording clinical symptoms was considered significant; for this reason, such cases are included in Table 28. We were able to demonstrate a significant midline shift of more than 2 mm in 15 out of 100 patients suspected of possessing a brain tumor. A supratentorial space-occupying lesion was subsequently confirmed in 10 cases (66.6%), and unilateral atrophy in a further 2 of these patients (13.3%). Midline displacement of 2 mm was exhibited in 2 of the 12 patients (18.3%) with a supratentorial mass. A further 2 subjects with a mass lesion above the tentorium revealed bilaterally synchronous midline echoes.

Demonstration of diencephalic shifts larger than 2 mm was possible in only 2 of the 8 patients with a confirmed infratentorial mass. Insignificant shifts under 2 mm or bilaterally corresponding midline echoes were demonstrated in the remaining 6 cases.

Abnormal expansion of the lateral ventricles was observed in 9 of the 12 cases (75%) with a confirmed mass above the tentorium. In contrast, all 8 patients (100%) possessing an infratentorial expanding lesion exhibited ventricular dilatation.

Midline shifts of 2 mm or more were exhibited by 8 of the 12 patients (66.6%) with a confirmed supratentorial mass, and by 2 of the 8 patients (25%) with an infratentorial lesion. From a total of 15 significant midline shifts, 8 patients (53.3%) ultimately revealed a mass lesion above, and 2 below, the tentorium.

The above comparisons are intended to demonstrate SEG limitations. We were able to correlate significant SEG shift and the presence of an intracranial mass in 66.6% of our cases. Therefore, isolated midline shift does not necessarily indicate the existence of a brain tumor, since displaced midline echoes toward the affected side occurred in various unilateral atrophical conditions. Case No. 10 and No. 11 should illustrate the above.

F. Comparison of SEG and EEG Findings

Table 29 relates the side to which midline structures were displaced in the SEG to the side on which the EEG focal abnormality was demonstrated.

A supratentorial space-occupying lesion could not be demonstrated in any patient with midline shift directed toward the side of the EEG focus. An atrophical lesion was ultimately demonstrated in both cases where SEG midline shift was directed toward the same side as the EEG focus (see Case No. 10).

In 10 patients with midline displacement less than 2 mm away from or toward the EEG focus, one patient subsequently revealed a brain tumor above the tentorium (Case No. 16). Another subject with identical findings was found to have cerebral atrophy (Case No. 12).

As can be seen from Table 29, the diagnostic value of a focal EEG finding increases proportionally to SEG midline displacement. Of 7 patients with midline shifts of more than 2 mm toward the side opposite the EEG focus, a mass lesion

Table 29. *SEG midline shifts in relation to lateral location of EEG foci*

SEG findings in reference to focus hemisphere		No. of cases	Supra-tentorial	Infra-tentorial	Cerebral atrophy	Other CNS disorders
Shift of more than 2 mm	toward EEG focus	2	0	0	2	0
	away from EEG focus	7	5	0	0	2
Shift of exactly 2 mm away from EEG focus		1	1	0	0	0
Shift up to 2 mm in either direction		10	1	0	1	8
Grand total		20	7	0	3	10
Percentage		100%	35%	0%	15%	50%

Table 30. *Summary of SEG and EEG findings in 100 patients suspected of possessing an intracranial space-occupying lesion*

EEG	SEG	Supra-tentorial	Infra-tentorial	Atrophy	Various neurological disorders
Focal change	Shift toward focus over 2 mm	—	—	2	—
	No shift or under 2 mm in either direction	1	—	1	7
	Shift of 2 mm away from focus	1	—	—	—
	Shift of more than 2 mm away from focus	5	—	—	2
Diffuse change	Shift over 2 mm	2	1	—	—
	Shift of 2 mm	1	—	—	—
	Less than 2 mm or no shift	—	6	—	1
Normal	Shift of 2 mm or more	1	1	—	1
	Shift under 2 mm	1	—	—	66
Total	100	12	8	3	77
Total No. with hydro-cephalus	26	9	8	1	8
Per-centage with hydro-cephalus	100%	75%	100%	33.3%	10.3%

above the tentorium was demonstrated in 5 of them (71.4%) (see Cases No. 9, 11, and 13 to 16).

EEG-SEG findings in the 100 subjects included in this series are summarized in Table 30.

Suspicion of an intracranial space-occupying lesion was subsequently disproven in 3 cases where the diencephalic midline was shifted up to 3 mm toward the side of the EEG focus, and in the 66 patients exhibiting a normal EEG and SEG (see Case No. 10).

By means of the EEG-SEG combined examination, it was possible to clinically detect all intracranial lesions producing morphological and/or electrical abnormalities.

An intracranial space-occupying lesion could not be demonstrated in any of the patients with focal EEG changes accompanied by SEG midline shift directed toward the side of the focus. Unilateral cerebral atrophy was ultimately revealed through further contrast procedures in all patients exhibiting this combination of findings. Epileptical seizures were present in intial clinical examination of all patients in this group.

Contrary to those patients demonstrating epilepsy, atrophy, and SEG shifts toward the affected side, 5 out of 7 patients (71.4%) with a focal EEG abnormality and a SEG shift away from the side of the focus ultimately revealed a supratentorial mass. When patients with midline shifts of 2 mm are included, the probability of such a lesion increases to 85.7%. These findings correlate with those from other authors such as SANDOK et al. Moreover, patients with diencephalic shifts less than 2 mm and an EEG focus on the opposite side must be kept under observation, since in 8 of these patients (12.5%) a supratentorial space-occupying lesion was found.

It can consequently be said that the midline shifts which usually would be considered within normal range (2 mm or under) must be considered abnormal when these are combined with an EEG focus. Such findings necessitate further neurological study.

The extent of midline shift is closely correlated with tumor location. Expanding lesions of the frontal, occipital, and parasagittal regions can be considered in "echo deaf" zones, since even relatively large tumors in these regions produce little midline shift. When an EEG focus appears in one of these regions, a normal SEG does not exclude the possibility of a supratentorial space-occupying lesion.

Infratentorial tumors deserve special consideration, since they usually produce neither midline shift in the SEG nor focal changes in the EEG. At most, diffuse slowing of the EEG is observed. In our series of 8 infratentorial tumors, an abnormally expanded ventricular system was observed in the SEG of all subjects (100%).

Various illustrative cases should elucidate the diagnostic possibilities of the combined EEG-SEG examination.

In summary, it can be said that the results of our combined EEG-SEG examination of 100 children suspected of possessing an intracranial space-occupying lesion lead to the following conclusions:

1. A usually normal midline shift (2 mm or under) in the SEG must be considered significant when an abnormal focus is found in the corresponding EEG.

2. An intracranial space-occupying lesion should always be suspected when the SEG midline shift is to the side opposite the EEG focus. This possibility increases with the extent of the shift.

3. A focus in the EEG and a midline shift directed toward the same side is a significant sign of atrophical change.

4. When no intracranial disorder is present, both examinations are normal.

The combined EEG and SEG examinations complement each another perfectly. Both can be performed quickly and in one session without any risk to the patient. Both examinations can be considered a tremendous diagnostical and differential diagnostical aid.

Illustrative Cases

Case No. 9

Karin H., $9^{5}/_{12}$ years old, File No. 1450, was admitted on Feb. 2, 1968, because of vomiting, exhaustion and headache of unknown etiology.

Case History: No birth complications reported, inconspicuous development during early childhood, supposedly never seriously ill. Present complications began 3 days before admission.

Condition on Admission: No internal findings. Sedimentation rate 5/9. Acetone two plus.

Dismission: on Feb. 14, 1968.

After temporary improvement, repeated headache and vomiting. Repeated attacks of anesthesia in the left arm and transient aphasia lead to the second admission.

Second Admission on March 2, 1968.

Condition on Admission: Sedimentation rate 10/25.

Neurological Status: Mild paresis of the mouth branch of the right facial nerve, right, abducens paresis, right, latent hemiparesis corresponding reflexes in the extremities. Gait deviating to the left with general hesitation.

Ophthalmological Examination: Diplopia, visual field loss, partial hemianopsia, and papilledema in the right fundus of 2 and in the left fundus of $2^1/_2$ diopters.

EEG: Focus of slow wave activity with a maximum parieto-occipital (Fig. 45 A).

SEG: Distinct midline shift to the right. Diffuse microcystic reflections in the area of the left hemisphere to the midline (Fig. 45 B).

Evaluation: An EEG focus on the left side combined with tissue displacement to the right and additional reflections on the left in the SEG indicate a space-occupying lesion in the left hemisphere.

Carotid Angiography on the Left: Anterior cerebral artery displaced contralaterally. The medial group was elevated fronto-caudally.

Clinical Diagnosis: Tumor in the left temporal lobe.

Operation Findings: Expansive infiltrating tumor which occupied the left temporal pole was uncovered. The tumor, along with its profoundly penetrating extensions, was removed.

Anatomical Diagnosis: Malignant astrocytoma.

Dismission: June 7, 1968.

Karin demonstrated temporary improvement and even attended school. In spite of radiotherapy, recidivation occurred (Fig. 45 B). SEG and EEG became abnormal again.

Admission: Oct. 10, 1968, the child became increasingly somnolent, and expired on Dec. 12, 1968.

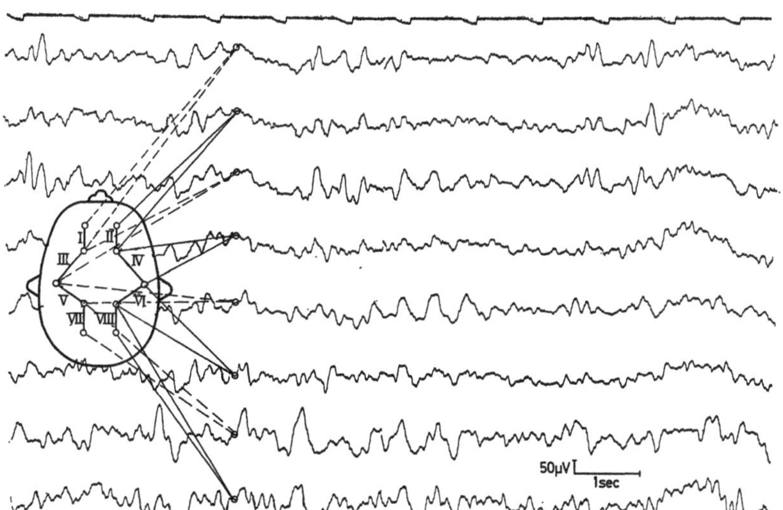

Fig. 45 A. Delta wave focus over the left hemisphere with a maximum in the parieto-occipital area

Alert EEG with eye closure from a $9^1/_2$ year old girl with a malignant astrocytoma in the left temporal lobe (Case No. 9, EEG No. 537/68, time constant 0.30, filter 70)

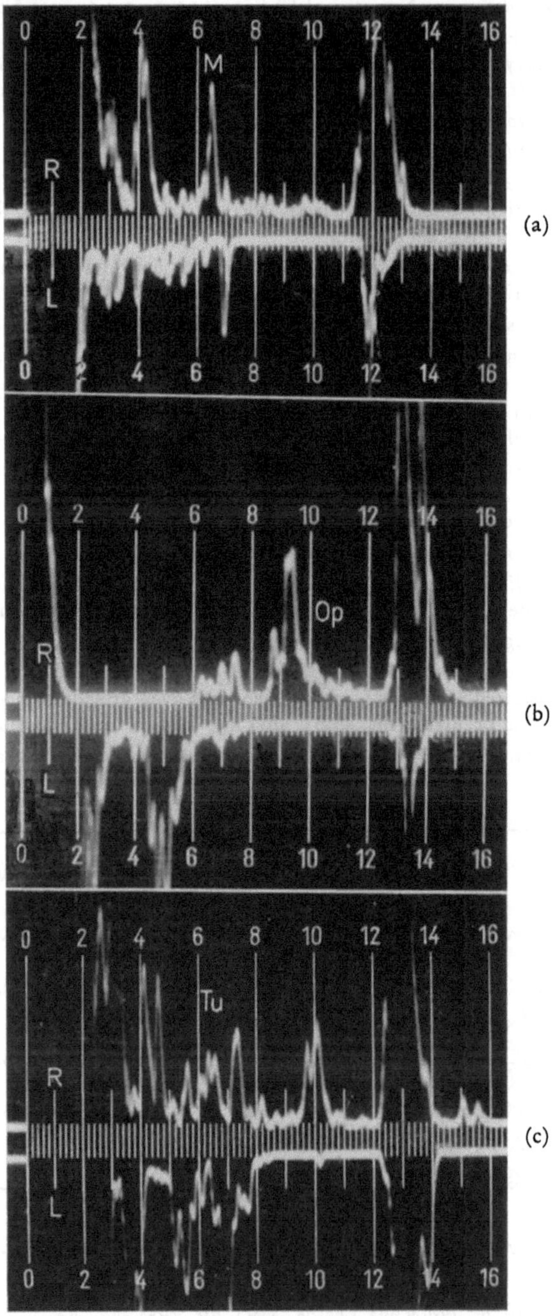

Fig. 45 B. Follow-up SEG examinations from Case 9. (a) Distinct midline shift of 4 to 4.5 mm toward the right side with diffuse microcystic reflections (tumor complex) in the left hemisphere, extending to the midline

(b) Extensive normalization (Op = operation site)

(c) Definitely abnormal sonoencephalogram with recurring tumor complex (Tu)

Case No. 10

Claudia C., $5^{2}/_{12}$ years old, File No. 5401, was admitted for diagnostic evaluation because of right-sided Jacksonian seizures.

Case History: Birth was without complications, weight 4500 g. Generalized convulsions for the first time at age 3 weeks. Normal mental and static development. Falling from a stool initiated seizures located on the right side. Intracranial hemorrhage was excluded by

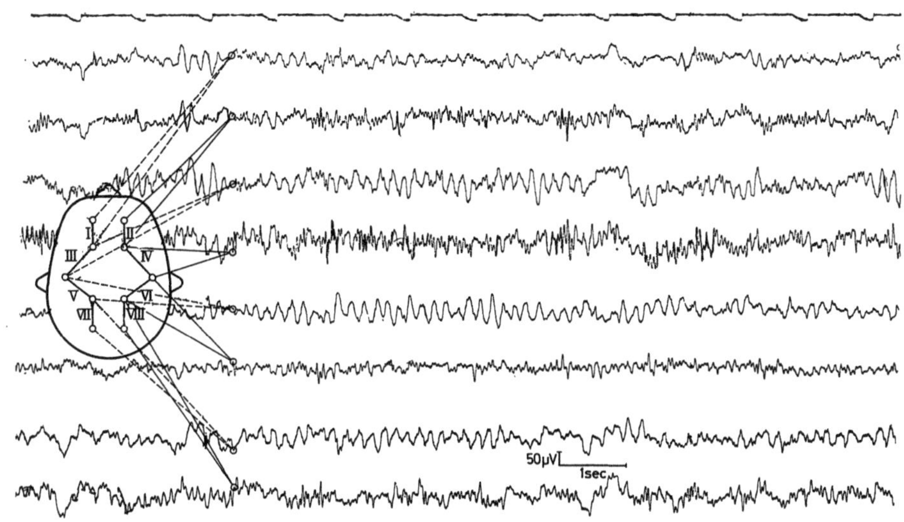

Fig. 46 a. A focus of monomorphic and polymorphic slow wave activity over the entire left hemisphere.
Alert EEG of a 5 year and 2 month old girl with cerebral atrophy on the left side (Case No. 10, EEG No. 423/69, t. c. 0.30/F 70)

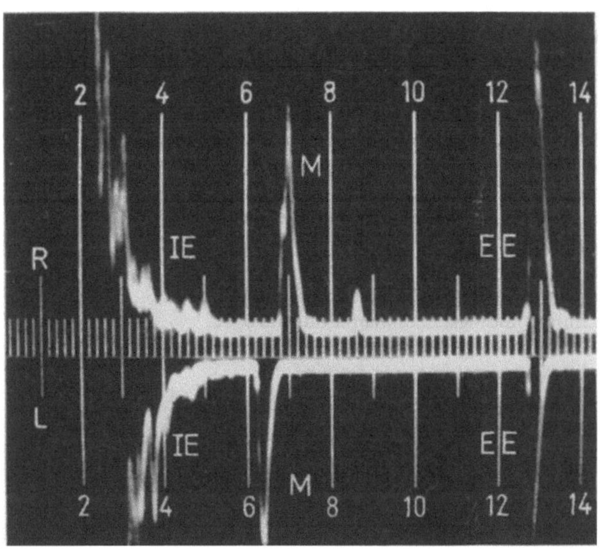

Fig. 46 b. Sonoencephalogram of the same patient with a shift of the midline structures of 3 mm toward the left side temporo-occipital trepanation on the left side. Since this time, the patient has suffered seizures lasting up to $2^1/_2$ hours occurring every $2^1/_2$ to $3^1/_2$ months. Antiepileptic therapy initiated.

Condition on admission: No abnormal internal findings.

Neurological Examination: With the exception of slight displacement of the tongue to the right, no cranial nerve abnormalities. Reflex and cerebellar function was intact. A mild muscular atrophy of the extremities on the right side was noticed. This was associated with motor limitation on the right side. Negative fundoscopy.

EEG: A focus of monomorphic and polymorphic slow wave activity was demonstrated over the entire left hemisphere (Fig. 46 a, p. 97).

SEG: Shift of the midline structures of 3 mm toward the left and a normal ventricular system were demonstrated (Fig. 46 b, p. 97).

Evaluation: A focus of slow wave activity over the entire left hemisphere in the EEG and tissue displacement towards the affected side in the SEG indicate cerebral atrophy in the left hemisphere.

Skull X-ray: Mild declination of the crista galli toward the left, deviation of the posterior sagittal suture to the left, and elevation of the superior border of the petrosum. The pneumoencephalogram was considered dispensable in this case.

Diagnosis: Cerebral atrophy on the left side of uncertain etiology.

Case No. 11

Anita C., $11^1/_{12}$ years old, File No. 6948, admission resulted from severe headache, vomiting and somnolence.

Case History: No known birth complications, development during early childhood reported to be normal. At age $10^8/_{12}$ years the child was taken ill with headache and temperatures up to 38.5 °C (101.3 °F), during which time she complained of extreme fatigue. This lead to admission in another clinic.

Neurological Status: Bilateral papilledema of 2 diopters. CSF demonstrated 3930/3 cells, mostly lymphocytes, sugar 48 mg%, protein 85 mg%, culture for microorganisms proved negative.

Diagnosis: Meningoencephalitis.

Therapy: Fluids and chloramphenicol.

Clinical Course: Cell number decreased rapidly: after 2 days, 1328/3; after the second-week of therapy, 250/3; and after the fourth week, 11/3. CSF protein value was at 105 mg%.

Fifth-Week of Therapy: EEG: Mild and diffuse slowing of wave activity. Neurological status: no basis for an expanding space-occupying lesion.

Eight-Week of Therapy: EEG: worsening of the previous findings. Neurological: papilledema unchanged. A 21-day prednisone therapy was initiated at this stage. Regression of the papilledema and normalization in the EEG was observed. After 12 weeks of treatment the patient was released at which time a further control admission was arranged.

Second Admission (14-weeks after first admission).

Neurological Status: Blurring of both optic disc margins. CSF cells 64/3. EEG: mild diffuse changes.

Third Admission (24-weeks after first admission).

Status: No clinical findings. Sedimentation rate 5/13.

Neurological: CSF 64/3 cells. Blurring of optic discs nasally on both sides.

EEG: Mild diffuse changes in wave activity.

Diagnosis: Chronic lymphocytic meningoencephalitis.

Fourth Admission (12 months after first admission): $12^1/_{12}$ years old, no clinical findings, CSF 26/3 cells, culture negative, sedimentation rate 5/14.

Neurological Status: Blurring of both optic disc margins.

EEG: Moderate diffuse changes in wave activity.

Skull X-ray: Signs of increased intracranial pressure.

Diagnosis on Discharge: Chronic lymphocytic meningoencephalitis.

Fifth Admission: History: The child was supposedly without complications until shortly before admission. A hesitant gait was observed 14 days before admission; vomiting and head-

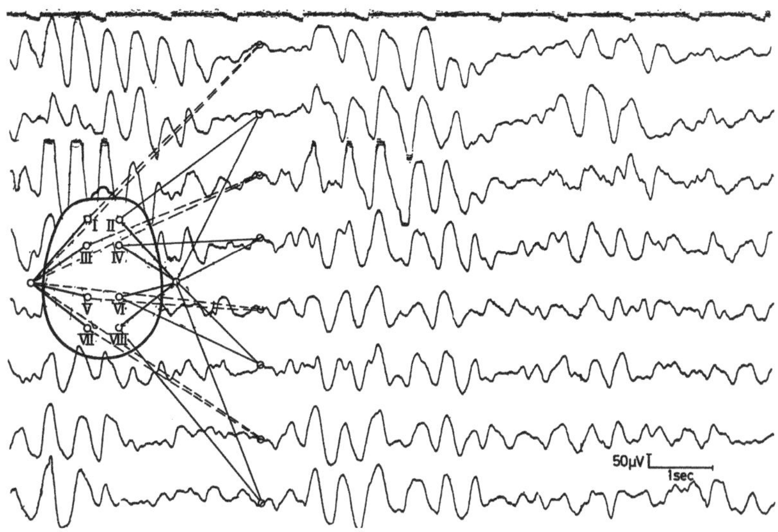

Fig. 47 A. Moderate diffuse changes in the form of slow wave activity
EEG of a 12 year old girl with an atypical ependymoma partially positioned within the right lateral ventricle (Case No. 11, EEG No. 1959/69, t. c. 0.30/F 70)

ache appeared 3 days before admission; loud crying during the night previous to admission. Transfer to our clinic.

Condition on Admission: This 12 year old girl exhibited fluctuating levels of consciousness, repeated vomiting, and complaints of headache. No abnormal internal findings, blood sedimentation rate after Westgreen 21/50.

Neurological Status: Obvious meningismus, increased reflexes on the left side, bilateral papilledema of 3 diopters. CSF findings: No. of cells 56/3, sugar 70 mg⁰/₀, protein 72 mg⁰/₀.

Skull X-ray: Signs of increased intracranial pressure.

EEG: Moderate diffuse changes of slow wave activity (Fig. 47 A).

SEG: Midline echo complex shifted to the left; lateral ventricular index 0.44, distinct ventricular dilatation (Fig. 47 B, p. 100).

Evaluation: Moderate diffuse alterations in the EEG, the expanded and shifted midline complex, and distinctly enlarged lateral ventricles indicate a tumor in the basal region.

Further Neurological Examinations: Brain scintiscanning exhibited positive findings in the form of a circumscribed area of radioactive activity on the parietal sagittal line.

Air Encephalogram: Internal hydrocephalus of the lateral ventricles accentuated on the right side and displacement to the left. Caudally displaced third ventricle and shift to the left.

Clinical Diagnosis: Space-occupying lesion in the area of the right lateral ventricle with mild structural displacement to the left.

Operation Findings: On Sept. 11, 1969, a partially intraventricular tumor was removed from the right hemisphere in toto, which was about the size of an apple.

Anatomical Diagnosis: Atypical ependymoma.

Case No. 12

Peter B., 20 months old, File No. 3247, was admitted for diagnostic evaluation of seizures and retardation of psychomotoric development.

Case History: Birth about 8 weeks premature, birth weight 2450 g. Post-partum signs of an asphyctic syndrome. During further progression, obvious retarded development and "cerebral" seizures.

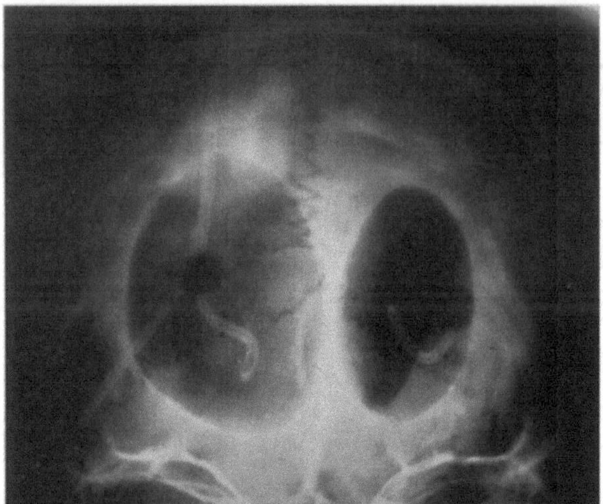

(a)

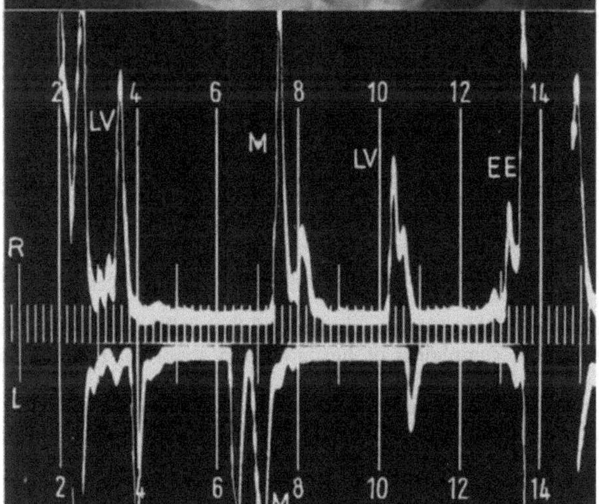

(b)

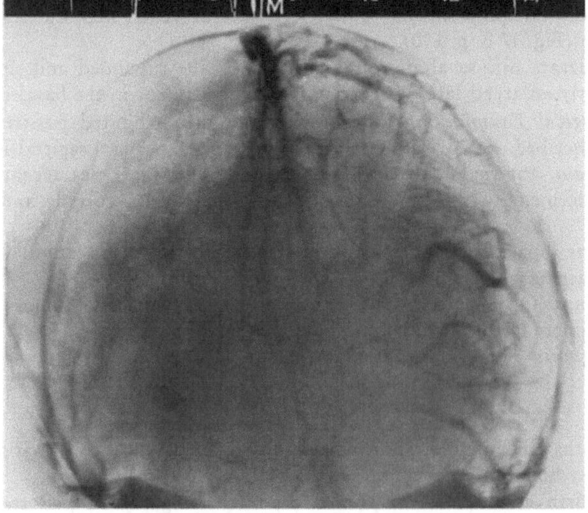

(c)

Fig. 47 B. Sonoencephalogram (b) from the same patient (Case No. 11) demonstrating displacement of the midline echo complex of 5 mm to the left and definite lateral ventricular dilatation (LVI = 0.44). Total agreement with pneumoencephalogram (a) and angiogram (c)

Condition on Admission: Small child, restricted in motion, does not sit or stand. No abnormal internal findings.

Neurological Status: Hypertony of the musculature, tetraspastic on the left side with increased reflexes. No papilledema and no abnormalities in the CSF.

EEG: Focus of slow wave activity and amplitude depression over the right hemisphere (Fig. 48 a).

SEG: Mild midline echo displacement to the right and considerable additional reflections (Fig. 48 b, p. 102).

Evaluation: EEG focus over the right hemisphere and a SEG midline shift toward the side of the focus indicate an atrophical lesion on the right side.

PEG: Cerebral atrophy on the right side was verified by demonstration of a large cavernous area filled with air. This was in the right hemisphere with a communication to the left lateral ventricle, which was slightly dilated (Fig. 48 b).

Diagnosis: Perinatal cerebral damage, tetraspastic, cerebral atrophy on the right side.

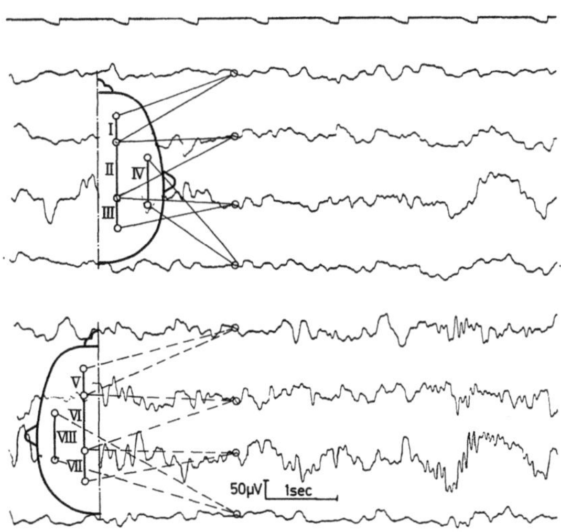

Fig. 48 a. Focal EEG findings in the form of slow theta waves and amplitude depression over the right hemisphere.
Sleep EEG of a 20 month old child with right-sided cerebral atrophy (Case No. 12, EEG No. 834/69, t. c. 0.30/F 70)

Case No. 13

Seglinde G., $18^{10}/_{12}$ years old, File No. 3162, was admitted because of headache, dizziness, vomiting, and focal seizures.

Case History: No birth complications reported. One of a set of twins. Development during early childhood normal. Two years ago a pseudotruncus arteriosus with a riding ventricular septum defect was diagnosed. Polycythemia. Two weeks before admission, the patient fell on the street and was unconscious for 15 minutes. During the following week she suffered several left-sided Jacksonian seizures, which were followed by paroxysmal hemiplegia with a decreasing tendency to return to normal.

Condition on Admission: Systolic murmur. Sedimentation rate 10/21.

Neurological Status: Psychomotoric development markedly retarded to that of about an 11 year old. Flaccid hemiplegia on the left, headache, dizziness, vomiting. Bilateral papilledema of 1 diopter in each eye.

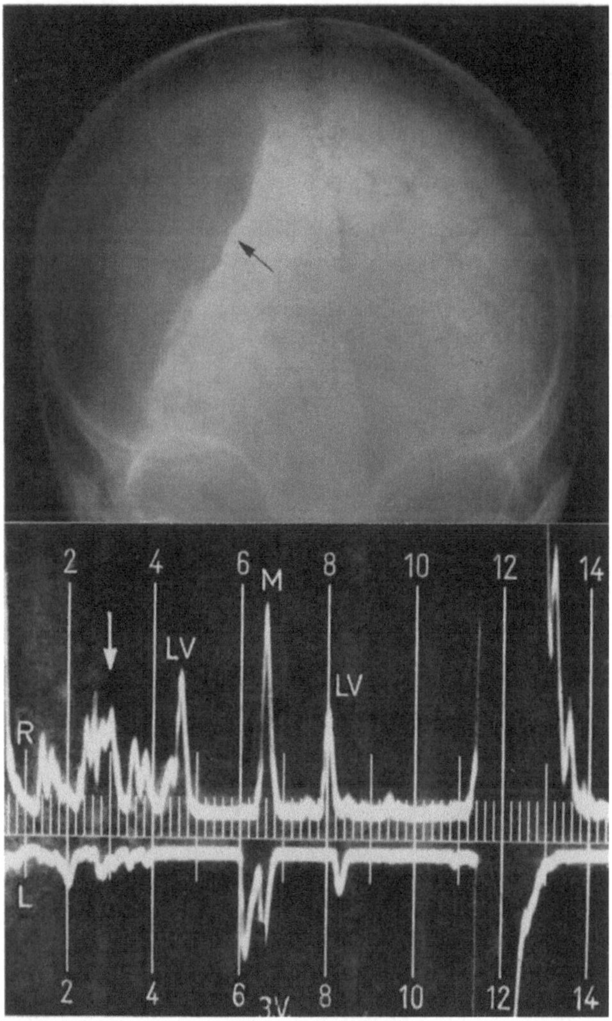

Fig. 48 b. Sonoventriculogram demonstrating additional reflections on the right side. This corresponds to right-sided atrophy observed in the PEG (indicated above with an arrow). The midline echo of this patient was found to be slightly shifted in the direction of the atrophical hemisphere (right) (Case No. 12)

EEG: Distinct focus of δ-waves on the right side with a maximum over the precentral region (Fig. 49 a).

SEG: Midline echo shift of 6 mm to the left and additional reflections on the right (Fig. 49 b). Total agreement with PEG and angiogram.

Evaluation: Space-occupying lesion in the area of the right hemisphere.

Carotid Angiography on the Right: Expansive lesion on the right extending from the parietal to the fronto-temporal region. Specific diagnosis: Most probably a cerebral abscess that has existed for a longer period and has developed vascularization on the capsulae wall.

Puncture: 10 ml of viscous pus was aspirated.

Evaluation: Arterial brain embolus originating from the known congenital cardiac anomaly associated with thickening of the blood and abscess development.

Diagnosis: Cerebral abscess.

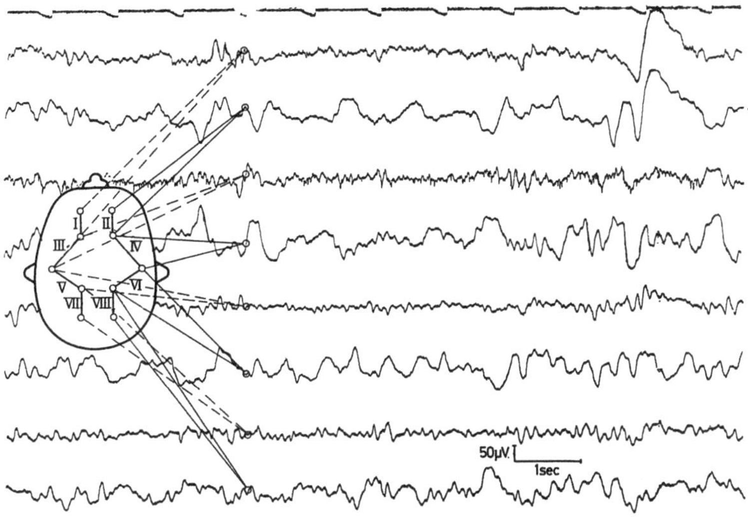

Fig. 49 a. Obvious focus composed of delta waves on the right side with maximum activity over the precentral region
Alert EEG of an $18^{10}/_{12}$ year old girl with a brain abscess on the right side and severe psychomotoric retardation (Case No. 13, EEG No. 717/69, t. c. 0.30/F 70)

Case No. 14

Ines-Martina K., $1^{5}/_{12}$ years old, File No. 8804, admitted because of increasing motor disturbance and refusal to eat.

Case History: Birth was reported without complications. Four hours post-partum the patient was observed experiencing apnotic seizures. The EEG demonstrated amplitude depression over the left parieto-occipital region which normalized after 12 days. Afterwards, normal development was reported.

At age one year the child first visited our outpatient clinic because of questionable seizures. She was reported to have suddenly jerked her arms and legs together, thereby exhibiting a fearful gaze.

At age $1^{3}/_{12}$ years increasing stiffness of the gait was noticed when the patient attempted to walk. The child became increasingly apathetic and forgot how to stand and sit within a short time. Within the last weeks it was observed that she could not sleep, refused to eat, and experienced nightly attacks of screaming.

Condition on Admission: No internal findings.

Neurological Status: Macrocephaly (1 cm above the 90th percentile) associated with depressed fontanelles. It was noticed that she could not sit or walk and that control of head movement was absent. Paresis of the facial nerve, reduction in movement of the right leg semilar to hemiplegia, and increased deep tendon reflexes on the right were observed as well. Papilledema was absent.

Skull X-ray: Open sutures.

EEG: Focus of delta wave activity over the left posterior area.

SEG: No midline echo shift, lateral ventricular dilatation (LVI = 0.49). The third ventricle could not be demonstrated because of numerous additional reflections in this area (Fig. 50, p. 105).

Evaluation: No corresponding SEG midline shift either toward the side of the EEG focus or in the opposite direction could be demonstrated. Dilatated lateral ventricles and additional reflections in the area of the third ventricle indicate a deep-seated intracranial space-occupying lesion.

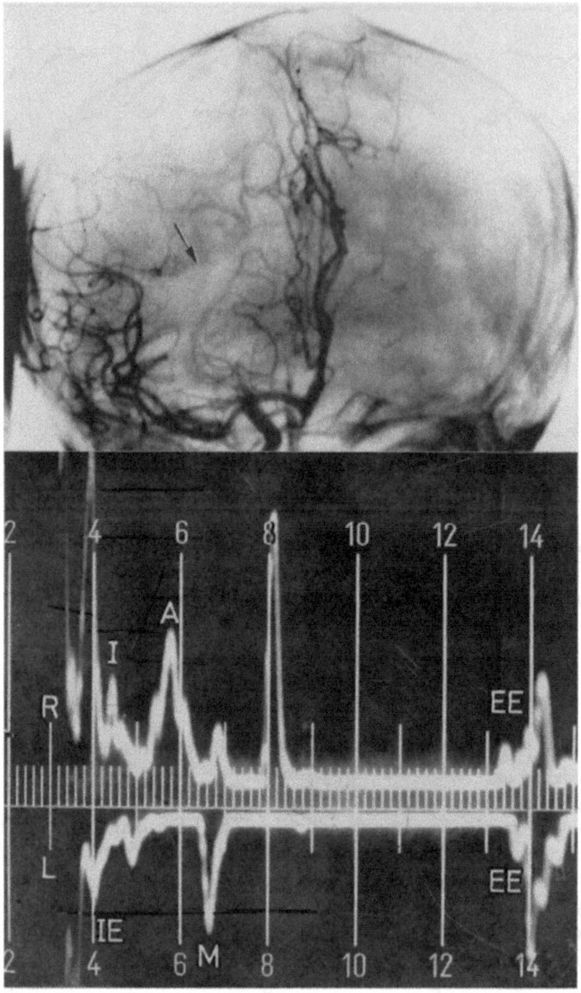

Fig. 49 b. Sonoencephalogram of the same patient demonstrating midline echo shift of 6 mm toward the left side and additional pyramid-like reflections (A) on the right side. These reflections appeared constant when beaming from the right side. Total agreement demonstrated in the angiogram (Case No. 13). The position of the abscess (A) is indicated with an arrow in the angiogram

Carotid Angiography on the Right: Anterior cerebral artery stretched. The medial group appeared lateralized, extended and stretched (Fig. 50 d, p. 105).

PEG: Occlusive hydrocephalus (Fig. 50 b, p. 105).

Findings on Operation: A tumor extending from the cerebellar vermis to both sides of the aqueduct was removed. Portions in the immediate area of the aqueduct were not disturbed. Tordildson drainage.

Anatomical Diagnosis: Ependymoma.

Clinical Course after Operation: Continuous radiotherapy. However, the child expired at age $1^{9}/_{12}$ years resulting from paralysis of the respiration control centers.

Post-mortum Findings: Recidivating tumor, internal hydrocephalus and cerebral edema.

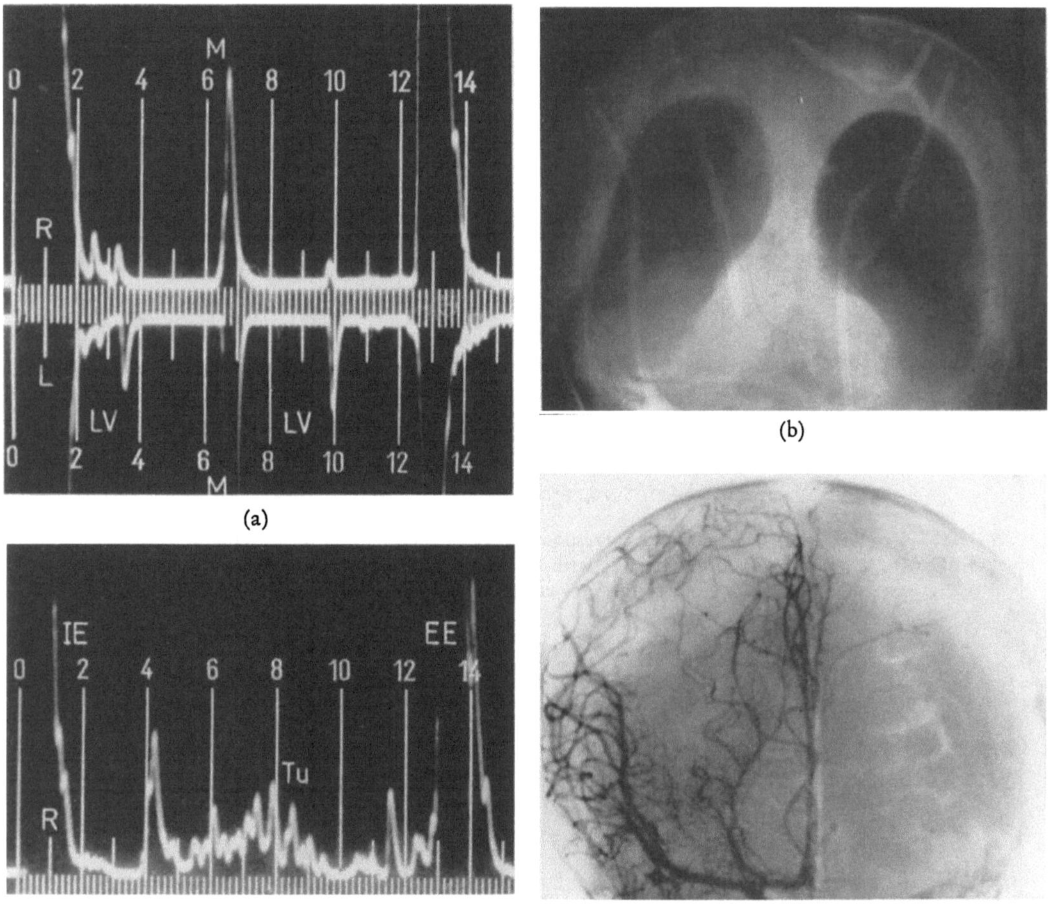

Fig. 50. No midline echo shift, enlarged lateral ventricles (a) (LVI $= \frac{64}{126+5} = 0.49$). Definite representation of third ventricular echoes is complicated by additional reflections from this area (c). Complete correlation with air encephalogram (b) and angiogram (d)

Case No. 15

Oswin R., $2^{1}/_{2}$ years old, File No. 1145, admitted because of headache and hesitating gait.

Case History: Birth was reported without complications. Normal development during early childhood. Since age three months, progressive hemiparesis with a hesitating gait. Severe headache within the last few weeks.

Condition on Admission: No abnormal internal findings. Sedimentation rate 3/11.

Neurological Status: In general, a very slow shild with flaccid hemiparesis on the left. Increased reflexes in the left extremities, uncertainty in grasping with the left hand and dragging of the left leg were also noticed. Papilledema was not observed.

Skull X-ray: Distension of the cranial sutures.

EEG: Basal activity corresponding to patient age. No focal abnormalities were demonstrated (Fig. 51 a).

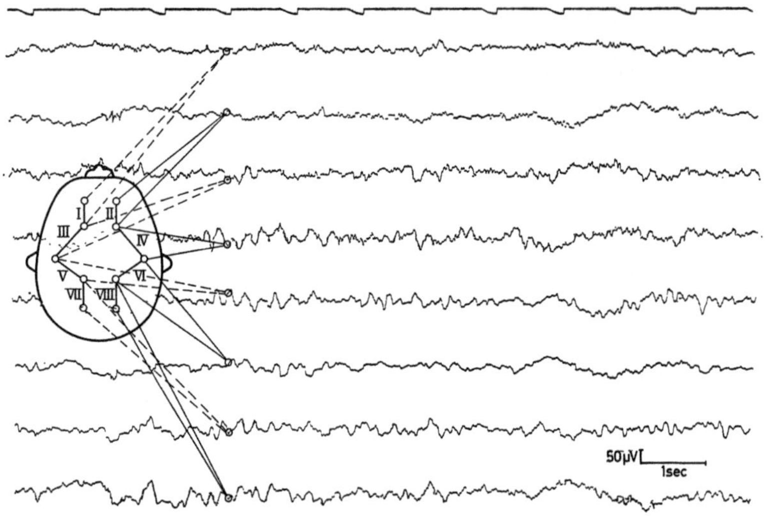

Fig. 51 a. Basal activity corresponding to patient age; no focal changes
EEG of a $2^5/_{12}$ year old drowsy child with an inoperable brain tumor (Case No. 15, EEG No. 214/68, time constant 0.30, filter 70)

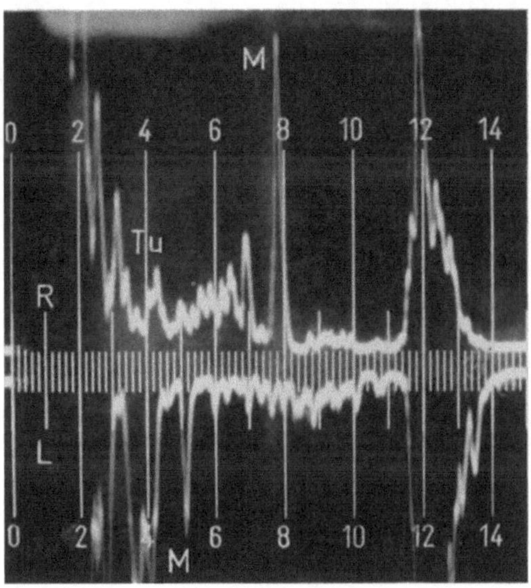

Fig. 51 b. Sonoencephalogram in the same patient. Distinct midline shift toward the left side with diffuse microcystic reflections in the right hemisphere extending to the midline (M). The third ventricle could not be clearly demonstrated because of tumor reflections (Tu) (Case No. 15)

SEG: Obvious displacement of the midline echo to the left and diffuse microcystic reflections on the left extending to the midline echo. The third ventricle could not be definitely demonstrated (Fig. 51 b).

Evaluation: Normal EEG, abnormal SEG with a shift to the left, and a tumor complex indicate neoplasmic growth on the right side. This combination of findings virtually excludes the cerebral cortex as a possible location of the tumor.

Carotid Angiography on the Right: The anterior cerebral artery was slightly displaced to the contralateral side. Severe convex elevation of the initial components of the medial group. The posterior cerebral artery was obviously displaced basally in its temporal portion.

Diagnosis: Tumor (approximately the size of a peach) in the area of the third ventricle.

Findings at Operation: Inoperable tumor in the midbrain. Placement of a ventriculo-auricular by-pass after Spitz-Holter.

Case No. 16

Martin K., $11^5/_{12}$ years old, File No. 9605, admitted because of headache, dizziness and vomiting.

Case History: Birth reported without complications. The patient complained of chronic fatigue. Two weeks before admission nausea in the morning, dizziness, and hesitation of the gait were reported.

Condition on Admission: Neurological: Apathetic, moderately slow boy with lively reflexes, meningismus, slight paresis of the facial nerve, and a broad atactic gait. Papilledema on the right with 3.5, on the left with 4 diopters.

EEG: Definite delta focus over the right frontal area (Fig. 52 a).

SEG: Slight midline echo shift of 2 mm to the left (Fig. 52 b). Ventricular system within normal limits.

Evaluation: An EEG focus over the right frontal region and slight midline displacement in the SEG in the presence of a normal ventricular system indicates a space-occupying lesion in the cerebral cortex.

Carotid Angiography on the Right: The superior cerebral artery was contralaterally displaced. The medial group was compressed in the area of the pars sphenoidalis.

Findings at Operation on Dec. 10, 1968: A fronto-lateral tumor (about the size of a tangerine) was removed in toto.

Histology: Malignant astrocytoma.

Discharge: On March 20, 1969.

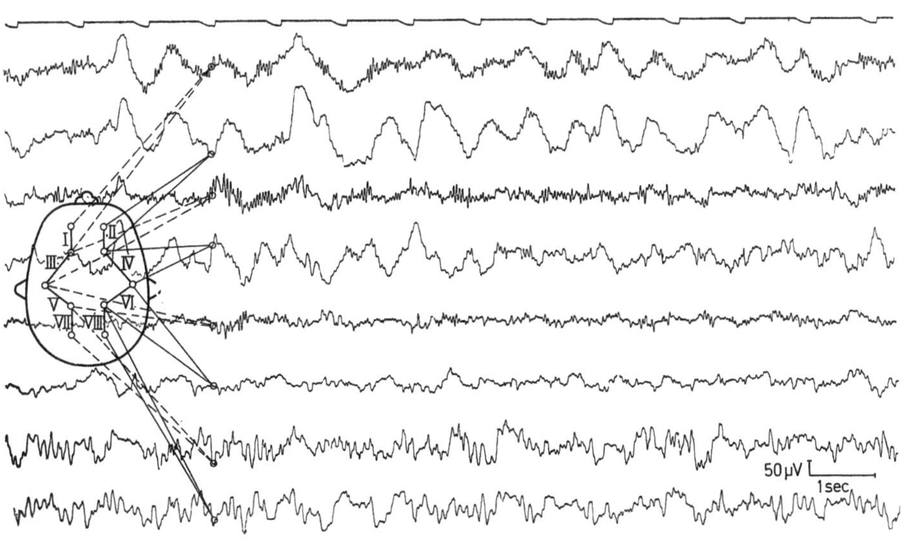

Fig. 52 a. Obvious delta focus over the right frontal lobe
Alert EEG of a $11^5/_{12}$ year old boy during eye closure. A fronto-lateral malignant astrocytoma was discovered (Case No. 16, EEG No. 217/68, time constant 0.30, filter 70)

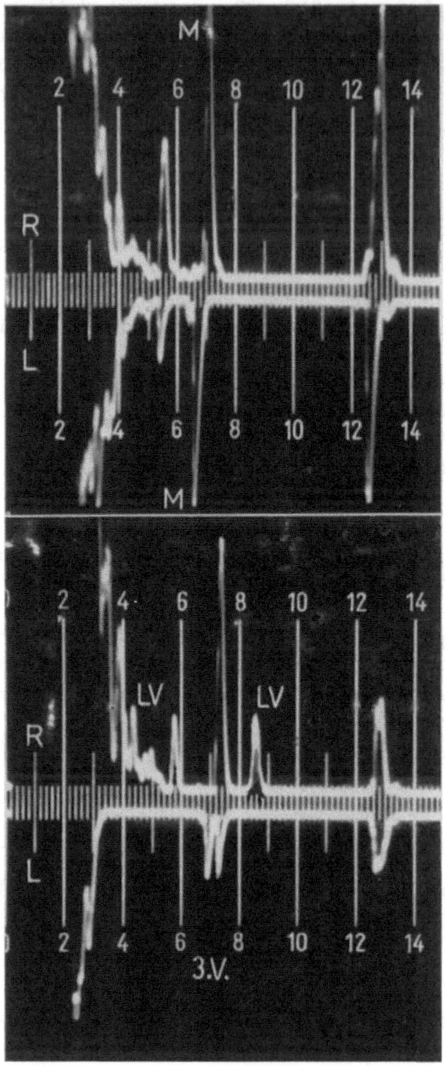

Fig. 52 b. Top: Mild midline shift of 2 mm which cannot be considered as definitely abnormal (Case No. 16). Bottom: Normal sonoventriculogram from the same patient. Abbreviations: M = midline echo, LV = lateral ventricular outer wall, and 3. V. = third ventricle

References

Abe, Y., Ohara, Y., Sato, K., Sugawara, K., Ito, K., Kikuchi, S.: Study on the shift of midline echo in the intracranial disease. Japan. Med. Ultrasonics **3**, 53 (1965).

— — Sugawara, K., Ito, K., Kikuchi, S.: Diagnostic value of the third ventricle echo in the case of head injury. Japan. Med. Ultrasonics **4**, 36 (1966 a).

— Sugawara, K., Ishii, M., Ito, K., Kikuchi, S., Tanaka, K.: Diagnosis of head injury by ultrasonic technique — Diagnostic values of hematom echo. Japan. Med. Ultrasonic **4**, 58 (1966 b).

— Tanaka, K., Wagai, T., Ito, K.: Diagnosis of intracranial hemorrhage using ultrasound. Acta radiol. **5**, diagnosis, 7th Symposium neuroradiol., New York 1964, 721—729 (1966 c).

Achar, V. S., Coe, R. P. K., Marshall, J.: Echoencephalography in the differential diagnosis of cerebral haemorrhage and infarction. Lancet **1966 I**, 161—164.

Adam, A.: Erste Versuche mit Ultraschallbehandlung im Kindesalter. Mschr. Kinderheilk. **97**, 391—393 (1949).

— Ultraschallbehandlung im Kindesalter. Ultraschall in Med. **I**, 247—277 (1949).

Adams, J. H.: Discussion of Achar, Coe and Marshall. Lancet **1966 I**, 487—488.

Adapon, B. D., Chase, N. E.: 'B' scan encephalography. Acta radiol. **5**, diagnosis, 7th Symposium neuroradiol., New York 1964, 730—739 (1966).

— — Kricheff, I. I., Battista, A. F.: Cerebral ultrasonic tomography. Radiology **84**, 115 to 121 (1965).

Ahrens, E.: Schall und Ultraschall in der Unterwasser-Nachrichtentechnik. Arbeitsgemeinschaft f. Forschung des Landes Nordrhein-Westfalen 101. Köln: Westdeutscher Verlag 1961, S. 47—77.

Akerman, M., Basso, A.: L'exploration cérébrale par une technique d'écho-B. Intérêt et limites. Neuro-chirurgie **13**, 527—536 (1967).

— Guiot, G.: Le diagnostic des processus expansifs intracraniens par l'association de la gamma- et de l'échoencéphalographie (Etude statistique de 650 cas). Ann. radiol. **8**, 851—879 (1965).

Allen, R. J., Gibson, R. M.: Phenylketonuria with normal intelligence. Amer. J. Dis. Child. **101**, 115 (1961).

Alvord, E., Stevenson, L., Vogel, R., Angle, R.: Neuropathological findings in phenylpyruvic oligophrenia (Phenylketonuria). J. Neuropath. exp. Neurol. **9**, 298 (1950).

Ambrose, J.: Some clinical applications of ultrasound. Brit. J. Radiol. **36**, 302 (1963).

— Pulsed ultrasound. Illustrations of clinical applications. Brit. J. Radiol. **37**, 165—178 (1964).

Anderson, G. V., Niswonger, J. W.: Cephalometry with ultrasound. Amer. J. Obstet. Gynec. **91**, 563—567 (1965).

Andrew, D. S.: Ultrasonography in pregnancy. An enquiry into its safety. Brit. J. Radiol. **37**, 185—186 (1964).

Avant, W. S., Jr.: Pulsatile echoencephalography. A review and the importance of the respiratory factor. Neurology (Minneap.) **16**, 1033—1040 (1966).

Bailey, O. T., Ingraham, F. D., Weadon, P. S., Susen, A. F.: Tissue reactions to powdered tantalum in the central nervous system. J. Neurosurg. **9**, 83—92 (1952).

Baldes, E. J., Herrick, J. F., Stroebel, Ch. F.: Biologic effects of ultrasound. Amer. J. phys. Med. **37**, 111—121 (1958).

Ballantine, H. T., Bell, E., Manlapaz, J.: Progress and problems in the neurological applications of focused ultrasound. J. Neurosurg. **17**, 858—876 (1960).

BALLANTINE, H. T., BOLT, R. H., HUETER, T. F., CAVALIERI, A., DYER, I., DOZOIS, E.: The detection of intracranial tumors by use of ultrasound. M. I. T. Acoust. Lab. Quarterly Progr. Report, Jan.—March (1951).
— — — LUDWIG, G. D.: On the detection of intracranial pathology by ultrasound. Science 112, 525—528 (1960).
— HUETER, T. F., BOLT, R. H.: On the use of ultrasound for tumor detection. J. acoust. Soc. Amer. 26, 581 (1954).
— — NAUTA, W. J. H., SOSA, D. M.: Focal destruction of nervous tissue by focused ultrasound. Biophysical factors influencing its application. J. exp. Med. 104, 337—360 (1956).
— LUDWIG, G. D., BOLT, R. H., HUETER, T. F.: Ultrasonic localization of the cerebral ventricles. Trans. Amer. Neurol. Ass. 75, 38—41 (1950).

BAMBERGER, PH., MATTHES, A.: Anfälle im Kindesalter. Basel-New York: S. Karger 1959.

BARROWS, H. S., DYCK, P., KURZE, T.: The diagnostic applications of ultrasound in neurological disease. Neurology (Minneap.) 15, 361—366 (1965).
— — — Reliability and limits of echoencephalography in acute neurological conditions. Intern. Symposium Echo-Encephalography. Erlangen 14./15. April 1967.
— KURZE, TH.: The value of ultrasonic encephalography as an adjunct to neurology and neurological surgery. In: Neurological diagnostic techniques. Ed.: W. S. FIELDS. Springfield (Ill.): Thomas 1966, pp. 1—29.

BARTH, G., BÜLOW, H. A.: Zur Frage der Ultraschallschädigung jugendlicher Knochen. Strah-Strahlentherapie 79, 271—280 (1949).
— PÄZOLD, J., WACHSMANN, F.: Über den Wirkungsmechanismus biologischer Ultraschallreaktionen. Strahlentherapie 80, 305 (1949).
— WACHSMANN, F.: Biologische Grundlagen der Ultraschalltherapie. In: Ultraschalltherapie. Hrsg.: R. POHLMAN. Bern: Huber 1951.

BARTHEL, R.: Sound velocity in some aqueous solutions as a function of concentration and temperature. J. acoust. Soc. Amer. 26, 227—230 (1954).

BAUER, B. L., GELETNEKY, C. L., LORENZ, R., SEEGER, W., VOGELSANG, H., WESEMANN, W.: Differentialdiagnose und Behandlung des akuten Koma. Aus neurologischer Sicht. Nervenarzt 37, 540—545 (1966).

BAUM, G.: A comparison of the merits of the scanned intensity modulated ultrasonography VS. Unscanned a scope ultrasonography. In: Diagnostic Ultrasound. New York: Plenum Press 1966.
— GREENWOOD, I.: The applications of ultrasonics locating techniques to ophthalmology. Theoretic considerations and acoustic properties of oculas media. Part I. Reflective properties. Amer. J. Ophthal. 46, 319—329 (1958).
— — The application of ultrasonic locating techniques to ophthalmology. Arch. Ophtal. 60, 263—279 (1958).
— — Ultrasonography—an aid in orbital tumor diagnosis. Arch. Ophtal. 64, 180—194 (1960).
— — A critique of time-amplitude ultrasonography. Arch. Ophtal. 65, 353—365 (1961).
— — Orbita lesion localization by three-dimensional ultrasonography. N. Y. St. J. Med. 61, 4149—4157 (1961).

BECHAR, M., BORNSTEIN, B., ELIAN, M., SANDBANK, U.: PKU presenting an intermittent progressive course. J. Neurol. Neurosurg. Psychiat. 28, 165 (1965).

BENDA, C. E.: In: Developmental Disorders of Mentation and Cerebral Palsies. New York: Grune and Stratton 1952, p. 451.

BERGMANN, L.: Der Ultraschall und seine Anwendung in Wissenschaft und Technik. 6. Aufl. Stuttgart: S. Hirzel 1954.

BERGSTRAND, C. G., BERGSTEDT, J., HERRLIN, K. M.: Pediatric aspects of brain tumors in infancy and childhood. Acta paediat. (Uppsala) 47, 688—705 (1958).

BERGSTROM, K., LODIN, H., SJÖGREN, I.: Echoencephalography and cerebral pneumography in infants and children. A comparative study with regard to ventricular size. 8e Symposium neuroradiol. Paris 1967.

BETZ, H., HUBER, G.: Zur Frage der Korrelierbarkeit von echoencephalographischen und pneumencephalographischen Befunden. Intern. Symposium Echo-Encephalographie. Erlangen 14./15. April 1967.

BICKEL, H.: Hirnatrophie und Störungen des Aminosäurestoffwechsels. Mschr. Kinderheilk. **115**, 254 (1967).
— GRÜTER, W.: Phenylketonurie mit normalen Intelligenzquotienten: Vergleichende biochemische und psychodiagnostische Untersuchungen von 2 etwa gleichaltrigen Mädchen. Z. Kinderheilk. **79**, 509 (1957).

BLATT, B.: Ekkoencefalografi med a-praesentation. Ugeskr. Læg. **128**, 1052—1056 (1966).

BLAUENSTEIN, U. W.: Die Ultraschallschnittbilduntersuchung im Oberbauch. Schweiz. med. Wschr. **99**, 985—992 (1969).
— PREISWERK, M., MÜLLER, H. R.: Physik, Technik und Terminologie der Ultraschalldiagnostik. Ultraschalltomographie. Arbeitstagung vom 15. März 1969 an der Chirurgischen Universitätsklinik Basel. (Vorsteher: Prof. M. ALLGÖWER.)

BLEIFELD, W., EFFERT, S.: Über den Nachweis cystischer Gebilde in verschiedenen Körperregionen mit dem Ultraschallreflexionsverfahren. Med. Wschr. **39**, 1747—1750 (1967).

BÖHMER, G., CARLSSON, C. A.: Entscheidende Faktoren für die Behandlungserfolge beim Epiduralhämatom. Mschr. Unfallheilk. **67**, 414—428 (1964).

BOLT, H., HUETER, T. F.: Some aspects of transcranial ultrasonic transmission. Ultraschall in Med. **6**, 202—203 (1953).

BRAAK, J. W., TER, CREZÉE, P., GRANDIA, W. A. M., DE VLIEGER, M.: The significance of some reflections in "Echo-Encephalography". Acta neurochir. (Wien) **9**, 382—397 (1961).
— GRANDIA, W. A. M., DE VLIEGER, M.: "Echo-Encephalography" as an aid in the diagnosis of subdural and extradural haematomas. In: Recent neurological research. Eds.: A. BIEMOND et al. Amsterdam: Elsevier 1959, pp. 37—45.
— DE VLIEGER, M.: Cerebral pulsations in echo-encephalography. Acta neurochir. (Wien) **12**, 678—694 (1965).

BRAHME, F., TRÄGER, B.: Echoencephalographic estimation of the size of the lateral cerebral ventricles in normal children. Radiology **92**, No. 1 (1969).

BRAUN, H., SCHMITT, W.: Erfahrungen mit der Ultraschallkardiographie in der Diagnostik von Mitralvitien. Materia Medica Nordmark **14**, 533—539 (1962).

BRENNER, H.: Ist die Ultraschall-Echo-Encephalographie ein Fortschritt in der Diagnostik frischer Schädel-Hirnverletzungen? Wien. klin. Wschr. **77**, 267—269 (1965).

BRINKER, R. A.: Ultrasound brain scanning utilizing the contact method. In: Diagnostic Ultrasound. Eds.: C. C. GROSSMANN et al. New York: Plenum Press 1966, pp. 186—190.
— Simultaneous presentation echoencephalography. Radiology **88**, 360—361 (1967).
— KING, D. L., TAVERAS, J. M.: Echoencephalography. Amer. J. Roentgenol. **93**, 781—790 (1965).
— TAVERAS, J. M.: Ultrasound cross-sectional pictures of the head. Acta radiol. **5**, diagnosis, 7th Symposium neuroradiol., New York 1964, 745—753 (1966).

BROCKHOFF, V., KAZNER, E., SCHIEFER, W.: Die Kombination von Echo-Encephalographie und Kontrastmittelmethoden in der Diagnostik raumfordernder Prozesse in der hinteren Schädelgrube. 8e Symposium neuroradiol. Paris 1967.

BRONSON, N. R.: Techniques of ultrasonic localization and extraction of intra- and extraocular foreign bodies. Amer. J. Ophthal. **60**, 596 (1965).

BROWN, R. E.: A standardized procedure for echoencephalography and for analyzing echoencephalograms. Canad. med. Ass. J. **96**, 1349—1354 (1967).

BRÜCKNER, H.: Die Bedeutung der Echo-Encephalographie für Diagnose und Behandlung der subduralen Haematome. Beitr. Neurochir. **8**, 180—191 (1964).
— Die Echoencephalographie. Möglichkeiten und Grenzen der Methode. Helfen Heilen 44 bis 50 (1965).
— Der kindliche Hydrocephalus und seine Behandlung. Helfen Heilen 52—55 (1965).
— Die postoperativen Komplikationen im Echoenzephalogramm. Acta neurochir. (Wien) **13**, 578—579 (1965).
— KAZNER, E.: Die Diagnose intrakranieller Prozesse mit der Echoencephalografie. SRW-Nachr. **21**, 1—7 (1963).

BRÜSCHKE, G.: Tierexperimentelle Untersuchungen zur Frage der Schädigung von Testis, Ovar und gravidem Uterus durch Ultraschall. Z. ges. inn. Med. **10**, 895—899 (1955).

BRYLSKI, J. R., IZENSTARK, J. L.: Anatomic localization of midline echo in sonogram of the brain. Amer. J. Roentgenol. **93**, 811—815 (1965).

BULL, J. W. D., MARSHALL, J., SHAW, D. A.: Cerebral angiography in the diagnosis of the acute stroke. Lancet **1960 I**, 562—565.

BUSCHMANN, W.: Acoustic illusions in ophthalmic ultrasonography. Amer. J. Ophthal. **57**, **57**, 461—466 (1964).

— Probleme und Fortschritte der Ultraschalldiagnostik am Auge. Klin. Mbl. Augenheilk. **144**, 321—347 (1964).

— Zur Diagnostik der Carotisthrombose. Albrecht v. Graefes Arch. Ophthal. **166**, 519 bis 529 (1964).

CALATAYUD-MALDONADO, V., GELETNEKY, C, LORENZ, R.: Posibilidades de diagńostico con el ecoencefalograma. Arch. Fac. Med. Zaragoza **13**, 61—83 (1965).

— — — El ecoencefalograma. Nuveo medio de diagńostico en neurocircurgia. Recio. Rev. Col. Med. Prov. Ciudadreal. **3**, 25—36 (1966).

CAMPBELL, J. B., WEAVER, E. N.: The use of echo-encephalography in neurologic diagnosis. Sth. med. J. (Bgham, Ala.) **58**, 782—787 (1965).

CARLIN, B.: Ultrasonics. New York: MacGraw-Hill Book Co. 1960.

CARSTENSEN, E. L.: Measurement of the dispersion of velocity of sound in liquids. J. acoust. Soc. Amer. **26**, 858—861 (1954).

— LI, K., SCHWAN, H. P.: Determination of the acoustic properties of blood and its components. J. acoust. Soc. Amer. **25**, 286—289 (1953).

— SCHWAN, H. P.: Acoustic properties of blood and its components. In: Ultrasound in biology and medicine. Ed.: E. KELLY. Washington: Amer. Inst. Biol. Scienc. 1957, pp. 1—14.

CHADDUCK, W. M., CRUTCHFIELD, W. G.: Extracranial masses complicating the interpretation of echoencephalograms. A new technique for quantitative evaluation. J. Neurosurg. **21**, 699—703 (1964).

CHAPTAL, J., GROS, CL., JEAN, R., CAMPO, CL., BARJON, R.: Sur les tumeurs cérébrales de l'enfant, à propos de 14 cas. Arch. franç. Pédiat. **11**, 657—659 (1954).

CH'EN, K.-P., P'AN, Y.-H.: Intercerebral ultrasonic exploration. Chin. med. J. **83**, 506—510 (1964).

— — Preliminary report in the use of ventricular needle from lateral emission type ultrasonic probe for intracranial exploration. Zhong. Waike. Z. (Peking) **12**, 261—264 (1964).

CHRISTIAN, W.: Klinische Electroencephalographie. Stuttgart: Thieme 1969.

COATES, S., NORMAN, A. P., WOOLF, L. I.: Phenylketonuria with normal intelligence and Gowers' musculatur dystrophy. Arch. Dis. Childh. **32**, 313 (1957).

COBB, W. A.: The EEG of specific lesions. In: Encephalography. Eds. D. HILL and G. PARK. London: Macdonald 1963, 2. Aufl.

COE, R. P. K., MARSHALL, J.: Echoencephalography. Lancet **1966, I**, 430.

COHEN, P., KOZINN, P.: Phenylpyruvic oligophrenia in a jewish child. J. Pediat. **34**, 76 (1949).

COLOMBATI, S., PETRALIA, S.: Assorbimento di ultrasoni in tessuti animali. Ricerca Scientifica **20**, 71—78 (1950).

CORSELLIS, J. A. N.: The pathological report of a case of phenylpyruvic oligophrenia. J. Neurol. Neurosurg. Psychiat. **16**, 139 (1953).

CRAWFORD, A. E.: Ultrasonic engineering. London: Butterworth 1955.

— In: Echoencephalographie. Hrsg.: Zit. nach E. KAZNER, ST. KUNZE und W. SCHIEFER (1965).

CROME, L., PARE, C. M. B.: Phenylketonuria. A review and report of the pathological findings in 4 cases. J. ment. Sci. **106**, 862 (1960).

CUNEO, H. M., RAND, C. W.: Brain tumors in childhood. Springfield (Ill.): Thomas 1952.

DALSGAARD-NIELSEN, T.: Some clinical experience in the treatment of cerebral apoplexy (1000 cases). Acta psychiat. scand. Suppl. **108**, 101—119 (1956/57).

DALY, D., WHELAN, J. L., BICKFORD, R. G., MACCARTY, C. S.: The electroencephalogram in cases of tumors of the posterior fossa and third ventricle. Electroenceph. clin. Neurophysiol. **5**, 203—210 (1953).

DAVIDOFF, L.-M., DYKE, C. G.: The normal encephalogram. Philadelphia: Lea & Febiger 1969.

DELIUS, P.: Ultraschall in der medizinischen Diagnostik. Elektromedizin 9, 43—45 (1964).
DENIER, A.: Les ultrasons, leurs applications au diagnostic: Ultra-sonoscopie, et à la thérapeutique: Ultra-sonothérapie. J. Radiol. Electrol. 27, 481—487 (1946).
DENIER VAN DER GON, J. J., DUINHOUWER, J. C., MOLIN, C. E., DE VLIEGER, M.: Equipment for two-dimensional echoencephalography. Neurology (Minneap.) 16, 927—933 (1966).
— MOLIN, C. E., DE VLIEGER, M.: Comparison of scan techniques in two-dimensional echoencephalography. In: Diagnostic ultrasound. Eds.: C. C. GROSSMAN et al. New York: Plenum Press 1966, pp. 155—165.
DILLING, H., FEUERLEIN, W.: Altersbedingte Unterschiede in der echoencephalographischen Darstellbarkeit der medianen Hirnstrukturen. Arch. Psychiat. Nervenkr. 209, 404—414 (1967).
DISTEL, L., KASPER, W.: Das Echo-Encephalogramm beim Hydrocephalus und Subduralerguß im Kindesalter. Intern. Symposium Echo-Encephalographie. Erlangen 14./15. April 1967.
— NEUHÄUSER, G., SCHUCH, A.: Echoencephalographie im Kindesalter, Indikationen und charakteristische Befunde. Fortschr. Med. 87. Jg., Nr. 3 (1969).
DONALD, I., MACVICAR, J., BROWN, T. G.: Investigation of abdominal masses by pulsed ultrasound. Lancet **1958 I**, 1188—1195.
— BROWN, T. G.: Demonstration of tissue interface within the body by ultrasonic echo sounding. Brit. J. Radiol. **34**, 539—545 (1961).
DOTT, N. M.: Brain movement and time. Brit. med. J. **1960 II**, 12—16.
DREESE, M. J., HAYES, G. J., KEMPF, L. G.: Evaluating intracranial hematoma by echo EG. Acta radiol. 5, diagnosis, 7th Symposium neuroradiol., New York 1964, 767—773 (1966).
— — — The value of an A-mode echoencephalogram display. Neurology (Minneap.) **16**, 355—358 (1966).
— McGEE, F. E., HARRELSON, A. B.: Correlative aids in B-scan echoencephalography. Neurology (Minneap.) **16**, 766—770 (1966).
— McHENRY, L. C.: Studies of echo-EG correlations. Neurology (Minneap.) **14**, 271—272 (1964).
— NETSKY, M. G.: The clinical use of echo-encephalography. Virginia med. Mth. **90**, 539 to 548 (1963).
— — Studies of lateral reflections in the echoencephalogram. Neurology (Minneap.) **14**, 521—528 (1964).
— SUTER, C. G., RENNIE, L. E.: Two-dimensional echoencephalography ("B-scan"): Description of a modified horizontal plane found clinically useful. Intern. Symposium Echo-Encephalographie. Erlangen 14./15. April 1967.
DUGDALE, L. M.: Echo-encephalography: The use of pulsed ultrasound in neurological diagnosis. Aust. Radiol. **10**, 207—216 (1966).
DUMERMUTH, G.: Elektroencephalographie im Kindesalter. Einführung und Atlas. Stuttgart: Thieme 1965.
DUSSIK, K. TH.: Über die Möglichkeit, hochfrequente mechanische Schwingungen als diagnostisches Hilfsmittel zu verwerten. Z. ges. Neurol. Psychiat. **174**, 153—168 (1942).
— Ultraschall-Diagnostik, insbesondere bei Gehirnerkrankungen, mittels Hyperphonographie. Z. phys. Ther. **1**, 140—145 (1948).
— Zum heutigen Stand der medizinischen Ultraschallforschung. Wien. klin. Wschr. **61**, 1—8 (1949).
— Ultraschallanwendung in der Diagnostik und Therapie der Erkrankungen des zentralen Nervensystems. In: Der Ultraschall in der Medizin. Hrsg.: K. MATTHES und W. RECH. Zürich: Hirzel 1949, S. 283—287.
— Weitere Ergebnisse der Ultraschalluntersuchung bei Gehirnerkrankungen. Acta neurochir. (Wien) **2**, 379—396 (1952).
— Entwicklung und Aussichten der Ultraschall-Diagnostik mittels Durchschallung. Ultraschall in Med. **6**, 203—204 (1953).
— Probleme der Ultraschallanwendung in der Therapie der Erkrankungen des Zentralnervensystems. Ultraschall in Med. **6**, 159—162 (1953).
— The ultrasonic field as a medical tool. Amer. J. phys. Med. **33**, 5—20 (1954).
— DUSSIK, F., WYT, L.: Auf dem Wege zur Hyperphonographie des Gehirns. Wien. med. Wschr. **97**, 425—428 (1947).

DYCK, P., BARROWS, H. S., KURZE, T.: Echoencephalographic localization of subcortical tumors through the dura at the time of operation. Intern. Symposium Echo-Encephalographie. Erlangen 14./15. April 1967.
— KURZE, TH., BARROWS, H. S.: Intra-operative ultrasonic encephalography of cerebral mass lesions. Bill. Los Angeles neurol. Soc. **31**, 114—127 (1966).
EBERLE, H.: Das Echo-Encephalogramm bei Schädel-Hirn-Trauma. Praxis **53**, 1710—1714 (1964).
EDLER, I.: The diagnostic use of ultrasound in heart disease. Acta med. scand. Suppl. **308**, 32—36 (1955).
— The use of ultrasound as a diagnostic aid and its efforts on biological tissues. Continuous recording of the movements of various heart-structures using an ultrasound echo-method. Acta med. scand. Suppl. **170**, 9—65 (1961).
— GUSTAFSON, A.: Ultrasonic cardiogram in mitral stenosis. Acta med. scand. **159**, 85—90 (1957).
— HERTZ, C. H.: The use of ultrasonic reflectoscope for continuous recording of the movements of heart walls. Kung. Fysiogr. Sällskapets i Lund Förhandlingar **24**, 1—19 (1954).
— — Heart diagnostics by ultrasound. Stockholm Svensk Naturvetenskap 1961.
EFFERT, S., DOMANIG, E.: Diagnostik intraaurikulärer Tumoren und großer Thromben mit dem Ultraschall-Echoverfahren. Dtsch. med. Wschr. **84**, 6—8 (1959).
— ERKENS, H., GROSSE-BROCKHOFF, F.: Über die Anwendung des Ultraschall-Echoverfahrens in der Herzdiagnostik. Dtsch. med. Wschr. **82**, 1253—1257 (1957).
ELIZONDO-MARTEL, G., GERSHON-COHEN, J.: Medical ultrasonics. Essentials of echoencephalography. Amer. J. Roentgenol. **93**, 791—802 (1965).
ENGESET, A., LÖNNUM, A.: Third ventricles of 12 mm width or more. Preliminary report. Acta radiol. (Stockh.) **50**, 5—11 (1958).
— SKRAASTAD, E.: Methods of measurement in encephalography. Neurology (Minneap.) **14**, 381—385 (1965).
ESCHE, R.: Untersuchungen zur Ultraschallabsorption in tierischen Geweben und Kunststoffen. Acustica 1—2, Beih. 2, 71—74 (1952).
EVANS, W. A., JR.: An encephalographic ratio for estimating the size of the cerebral ventricles. Amer. J. Dis. Child. **64**, 820 (1942).
FALK, B., KIRSTEN, L., LÖFSTEDT, S., SILFERSKIÖLD, B.: Pneumo-encephalographic investigations in epilepsy. Acta psychiat. scand. **33**, 440—451 (1958).
FEIGENBAUM, H., WALDHAUSEN, J. A., HYDE, L. P.: Ultrasound diagnosis of pericardial effusion. J. Amer. med. Ass. **191**, 711 (1965).
FERREY, G.: Les applications diagnostiques des ultra-sons à la médecine. II. L'échoencéphalographie A. Ann. Radiol. **9**, 881—890 (1966).
FEUERLEIN, W., BACKMUND, H. U., FLIEGE, K.: Die Weite des 3. Ventrikels — Ergebnisse der vergleichenden Messung durch Echo-Encephalographie und Pneumencephalographie. 1st World Congress on Ultrasonic Diagnostics in Medicine, Wien 1969.
— Echoenzephalographie in der Chirurgie. Chir. Praxis **10**, 587—594 (1966).
— DILLING, H.: Zur Bestimmung des Mittelechos in der Echoencephalographie. Nervenarzt **36**, 401—403 (1965).
— — Die Echoenzephalographie. Med. Klin. **61**, 1061—1064 (1966).
— — Das Echo-Encephalogramm des 3. Ventrikels in verschiedenen Lebensaltern. Arch. Psychiat. Nervenkr. **209**, 137—147 (1967).
— — Das Echo-Encephalogramm des dritten Ventrikels in den verschiedenen Lebensaltern. Intern. Symposium Echo-Encephalographie. Erlangen 14./15. April (1967).
FINCHER, E. F., STREWLER, G. J., SWANSON, H. S.: The Torkildsen procedure. A report of 19 cases. J. Neurosurg. **5**, 213—219 (1948).
FIRESTONE, F. A.: Flaw detecting device and measuring instrument. USA-P. 2280226 (1940).
— Supersonic reflectoscope, an instrument for inspectious of the interior of solid parts by means of sound waves. J. acoust. Soc. Amer. **17**, 287 (1945).
FIRNHABER, W., DJAWDAN, M.: Das Echoencephalogramm als zusätzliche neurologische Untersuchungsmethode. Intern. Symposium Echo-Encephalographie. Erlangen 14./15. April 1967.
FISCHER, G., GERIN, P., REVOL, M., COURJON, J.: Place de l'écho-encéphalographie dans le diagnostic des lésions intracrâniennes. J. Méd. Lyon **46**, 85—102 (1965).

Fischer, G., Morin, A., Gerin, P., Courjon, J.: Aspects comparatifs des donnés écho- et électroencéphalographiques (A propos de 100 cas). Ann. méd.-psychol. **122**, 343 (1964).

— Revol, M., Munier, F., Gerin, P., Courjon, J., Wertheimer, P.: L'écho-encéphalographie. Valeur diagnostique et résultats. Neurochirurgía **10**, 45—58 (1967).

Fischgold, H.: Die Schädelunfall-Diagnostik. Dtsch. Röntgenkongreß 1965. Stuttgart: Thieme 1966, S. 126—130.

— Strauss, M.-F., Hazemann, P.: L'écho A dans les traumatismes du crâne. Intern. Symposium Echo-Encephalographie. Erlangen 14./15. April 1967.

Fliege, K., Backmund, H., Feuerlein, W.: Probleme und Ergebnisse bei der vergleichenden Messung des 3. Ventrikels durch Echoencephalographie und Pneumencephalographie. Arch. Psychiat. Nervenkr. **211**, 333—342 (1968).

Fois, A., Rosenberg, C., Gibbs, F. A.: The electroencephalogram in phenylpyruvic oligophrenia. Electroenceph. clin. Neurophysiol. **7**, 569 (1965).

Følling, A.: Über Ausscheidung von Phenylbrenztraubensäure in den Harn als Stoffwechselanomalie in Verbindung mit Imbezillität. Z. Physiol. Chem. **227**, 169 (1934).

Ford, R. M.: Echoencephalography—A method of determining frontal midline displacement. Inter. Symposium Echo-Encephalographie. Erlangen 14./15. April 1967.

— Ambrose, J.: Echoencephalography. The measurement of the position of midline structures in the skull with high frequency pulsed ultrasound. Brain **86**, 189—196 (1963).

— McRae, D. L.: Echoencephalography—A standardized technique for the measurement of the width of the third and lateral ventricles. In: Diagnostic ultrasound. Eds.: C. C. Grossman et al. New York: Plenum Press 1966, pp. 117—129.

Foster, J. J.: Ultrasonic encephalography. An aid in diagnosis of head trauma. J. int. Coll. Surg. **44**, 523—529 (1965).

Fox, J. L., Richards, J. R., Luessenhop, A. J.: Method for detecting intracranial arteriovenous malformation with an ultrasonic transducer using the Doppler phenomenon. J. Neurosurg. **26**, 322—326 (1967).

Fray, W. W.: Methods for determining pineal position with analysis of their errors. Amer. J. Roentgenol. **42**, 490—497 (1939).

Frankoni, G., Wallgren, A.: Lehrbuch der Pädiatrie. Basel/Stuttgart: Schwabe 1967.

French, L. A., Wild, J. J., Neal, D.: Detection of cerebral tumors by ultrasonic pulses. Pilot studies on post-mortem material. Cancer **3**, 705—708 (1950).

— — — The experimental application of ultrasonics to localization of brain tumours. Preliminary report. J. Neurosurg. **8**, 198—203 (1951).

Freund, H.-J.: Ultraschallregistrierung der Pulsation einzelner intrakranieller Arterien zur Diagnostik von Gefäßverschlüssen. Arch. Psyiat. Nervenkr. **207**, 247—253 (1965).

— Kapp, H.: Ultraschall-Echo-Registrierung arterieller Pulsationen in tiefen Körperregionen. Pflügers Arch. ges. Physiol. **289**, 96 (1966).

— — Eine Methode zur Registrierung arterieller Pulsationen mittels Ultraschall. Pflügers Arch. ges. Physiol. **291**, 268—276 (1966).

— — Kendel, K.: Arterielle Pulskurvenschreibung durch Ultraschall. Experimentelle Untersuchungen und diagnostische Möglichkeiten. Intern. Symposium Echo-Encephalographie. Erlangen 14./15. April 1967.

Friedman, G., Thun, F.: Zuverlässigkeit und Fehlermöglichkeiten der Echo-Enzephalographie bei supratentoriellen raumfordernden Prozessen. Med. Welt **50**, 689—696 (1964).

Friedrich, W., Mifka, P., May, V., Navratil, L.: Zur Frage des progredienten posttraumatischen Hydrocephalus internus. Wien. klin. Wschr. **75**, 826—828 (1963).

Frucht, A. H.: Die Schallgeschwindigkeit in menschlichen und tierischen Geweben. Z. ges. exp. Med. **120**, 526—557 (1952/53).

Fry, W. J.: Ultrasound in neurology. Neurology (Minneap.) **6**, 693—704 (1956).

— Use of intense ultrasound in neurological research. Amer. J. phys. Med. **37**, 143—147 (1958).

— Present and future applications of ultrasonics in biomedicine. Proc. Inst. Radio Engrs. **50**, 1393—1404 (1962).

Fuchs, P.: Die Bedeutung der Echo-Encephalographie bei der Beurteilung cerebraler Komplikationen Kieferverletzter. Fortschr. Kiefer- u. Gesichtschir. **11**, 112—115 (1966).

FUKUDA, T., TANAKA, K., et al.: Advance of Medical Application of Ultrasound developed by the Ultrasonic Research Group in Juntendo University Tokio 1964.

— WAGAI, T., TANAKA, K., et al.: Annual Report of the Medical Ultrasonic Research Center, Juntendo University Tokio 1965.

GALICICH, J. H., LOMBROSO, C. T., MATSON, D. D.: Ultrasonic B-scanning of the brain. J. Neurosurg. **22**, 499—510 (1965).

GELETNEKY, C.-L.: Echoenzephalographie im Säuglings- und Kindesalter. Acta neurochir. (Wien) **13**, 579—581 (1965).

— Die Bedeutung der Echoencephalographie für die Diagnostik und Verlaufskontrolle bei Tumoren der hinteren Schädelgrube. Vortrag Röntgenkongreß Baden-Baden 1967 (in press).

— Echoencephalographie bei cerebralen Erkrankungen im Säuglings- und Kindesalter. Acta radiol. 5, diagnosis, 7th Symposium neuroradiol. New York 1964, 779—785 (1966).

— KAZNER, E.: Die Echo-Encephalographie beim Hydrocephalus. Intern. Symposium Echo-Encephalographie. Erlangen 14./15. April 1967.

GERLACH, J., JENSEN, H.-P., KOOS, W., KRAUS, H.: Pädiatrische Neurochirurgie. Stuttgart: Thieme 1967.

GERLACH, W.: Physik. Frankfurt: Fischer 1960.

GIMENEZ, J. L., WINTERS, W. L., DAVILA, J. C., CONNELL, J., KLEIN, K. S.: Dynamics of the Starr-Edwards ball valve prothesis. A cine-fluographic and ultrasonic study in humans. Amer. J. med. Sci. **250**, 652 (1965).

GÖGLER, E.: Unfallopfer im Straßenverkehr. Basel: Documenta Geigy 1961.

GOHR, H., WEDEKIND, TH.: Der Ultraschall in der Medizin. Klin. Wschr. **19**, 25—29 (1940).

GOKALP, H., JAKOBY, R. K., WATTS, J. W.: Echoencephalography: An evaluation based on its use in 300 individuals. Med. Ann. D. C. **35**, 641—645 (1966).

GOLDBERG, B., ISARD, H. J., GERSON-COHEN, J., OSTRUM, B. J.: Ultrasonic Fetal Cephalometry. Proceedings of Radiol. Soc. Nth. Amer. Chicago 1965.

GOLDMAN, D. E., HUETER, T. F.: Tabular data of the velocity and absorption of high-frequency sound in mammalian tissues. J. acoust. Soc. Amer. **28**, 35—37 (1956).

GÖLLNITZ, G.: Über das normale Encephalogramm im Kindesalter. Nervenarzt **22**, 101—107 (1951).

GONSETTE, R., ANDRE-BALISEAU, G., COLLE, J.: Contribution de l'EEG au diagnostic des lésions de la fosse cérébrale postérieur (Revue de 131 cas vérifiés). Rev. Neurol. **95**, 530—537 (1956).

GORDON, D.: The use of ultrasonic rays in diagnostic radiology. Vortrag IV. Symposium neuroradiologicum. London 1955.

— Echoencéphalie. Rev. Neurol. **99**, 652—653 (1958).

— Echo-encephalography. Ultrasonic rays in diagnostic radiology. Brit. med. J. **5136**, 1500 to 1504 (1959).

— Echo-encephalography. In: Medical Electronics, proceedings of the second international conference on medical electronics. Paris 24—27 June 1959. London: Iliffe 1960, p. 380 to 390.

— Ultrasonic rays in diagnosis and surgery. Trans. med. Soc. Lond. **79**, 173—180 (1963).

— Ultrasound as a diagnostic and surgical tool. Edinburgh-London: Livingstone 1964.

— The limitations and uses of ultrasound in localizing cerebral lesions. Proc. roy. Soc. Med. **58**, 1053—1058 (1965).

— Ultrasonic surgery of the central nervous system. Acta radiol. 5, diagnosis, 7th Symposium neuroradiol., New York 1964, 796—803 (1966).

— Three-dimensional echo-encephalography in stereotaxic surgery. Intern. Symposium Echo-Encephalographie. Erlangen 14./15. April 1967.

— M. B., D. M. R.: Zwei- und dreidimensionale Ultraschalltechniken in der medizinischen Diagnostik. Schweiz. med. Wschr. **99**, 976—984 (1969).

GOTTESFELD, K. R.: The practical application of ultrasound in obstetrics and gynecology. In: Diagnostic Ultrasound. New York: Plenum Press 1966.

GREATOREX, C. A., IRELAND, H. J. D.: An experimental scanner for the use with ultrasound. Brit. J. Radiol. **37**, 179—184 (1964).

GREEBE, H. M.: De waarde van de echo-encefalografie als klinische en poliklinische methode van onderzoek. Ned. T. Geneesk. **108**, 10—13 (1964).

GROSSMAN, C. C.: Experience with combined EEG and ultrasound techniques in neurology. Neurology (Minneap.) **14**, 272 (1964).

— Clinical diagnostic application of ultrasound in brain disorders (sono-encephalography). Dis. nerv. Syst. **25**, 403—411 (1964).

— The normal sonoencephalogram (SEG). Ultrasonic echoes and brain structures. Dis. nerv. Syst. **25**, 717—723 (1964).

— Experience with combined EEG and ultrasound techniques in neurology. Neurology (Minneap.) **14**, 272 f. (1965).

— Acoustic phenomena in ultrasonic detection of brain tumors. Ultrasonics **3**, 22—24 (1965).

— EEG-SEG or soner. Ultrasonics **3**, 100—101 (1965).

— The use of diagnostic ultrasound in brain disorders. Springfield (Ill.): Thomas 1966.

— A- and B-scan sonoencephalography (SEG)—A new dimension in neurology. In: Diagnostic ultrasound. Eds.: C. C. GROSSMAN et al. New York: Plenum Press 1966, pp. 130 to 141.

— HOLMES, J. H., JOYNER, C., PURNELL, E. W.: Diagnostic ultrasound. Proceedings of the First International Conference, University of Pittsburgh 1965. New York: Plenum Press 1966.

GRÜTER, W.: Angeborene Stoffwechselstörungen und Schwachsinn am Beispiel der Phenylketonurie. Forum der Psychiatrie Nr. 5. Stuttgart: Enke 1963.

GURDIJIAN, E. S., THOMAS, L. M.: In: Davis, Christopher's Textbook of Surgery. Philadelphia-London-Toronto: W. B. Saunders Co., 9th Ed. 239 (1968).

GÜTTNER, W.: Betrachtungen zur Möglichkeit der US-Abbildung am menschlichen Schädel. Ultraschall in Med. **6**, 199—202 (1953).

— Die Energieverteilung im menschlichen Körper bei Ultraschall-Einstrahlung. Acustica **4**, 547—554 (1954).

— FIEDLER, G., PÄTZOLD, J.: Über Ultraschallbildungen im menschlichen Schädel. Acustica **2**, 148—156 (1952).

HACHE, H., SCHEID, P.: Das epidurale Hämatom. Pädiat. Prax. **5**, 415—422 (1966).

HATA, H., MARUTA, H., YOSHIDA, J., ISHIDA, K., INABI, Y.: Observation of hydrocephalus by ultrasound—Evaluation of effect of ventriculoauriculostomy. Japan. Med. Ultrasonics **2**, 41—43 (1964).

HEMMER, R.: Erfahrungen mit der modernen operativen Hydrozephalus-Behandlung. Beh. Arch. Kinderheilk. 51. Heft (1964).

— Über atypische posttraumatische epidurale Blutungen und die Ursachen ihrer Fehldeutung. Dtsch. med. Wschr. **90**, 1945—1948 (1966).

HENKE, G.: Ultraschall in der medizinischen Diagnostik heute. Elektromedizin **9**, 68—72 (1964).

HESS, R.: Misleading clinical and electrical signs in cerebral tumors. Electroenceph. clin. Neurophysiol. Suppl. **3**, 66 (1953).

— Electroencephalographische Studien bei Hirntumoren. Stuttgart: Thieme 1958.

— Elektrobiologische Phänomene bei erhöhtem intracraniellem Druck, Massenverschiebungen und Einklemmungen. 9e réunion européenne d'information électroencéphalographique. Marseille 12/13 oct. 1960.

— Significance of EEG-signs for location of cerebral tumors. Electroenceph. clin. Neurophysiol. Suppl. **19**, 75—110 (1961).

— Die bioelektrischen Zeichen der cerebralen Massenverschiebung bei Hirntumoren. Schweiz. med. Wschr. **92**, 1537—1542 (1962).

HILL, D., PARR, G.: Electroencephalography: A Symposium on its Various Aspects, Ed. 2. New York: The Macmillan Company 1963, p. 509.

HOFMANN, D., HOLLÄNDER, H.-J., WEISSER, P.: Neue Möglichkeiten der Ultraschalldiagnostik in der Gynäkologie und Geburtshilfe. Fortschr. Med. **84**, 689—693 (1966).

HOLMES, J. H., HOWRY, D. H.: Ultrasonic diagnosis of abdominal diseases. Amer. J. Dis. Child. **8**, 12—32 (1963).

HOLYST, J.: Zastosowanie ultradźwieków do badania organicznych zmian śródczaszkowych (echoencefalografia). Pol. Tyg. lek. **18**, 1109—1111 (1963).

— Echoencefalografia (Ultrasonoencefalografia). Pol. Tyg. lek. **18**, 1749—1752 (1963).

HÖPKER, W.: Die biologischen Wirkungen des Ultraschalls auf das Gehirn. Ultraschall in Med. **5**, 178—185 (1952).

HOTERMANS, J. M., THIRY, S.: L'échoencéphalographie—Examen préparatoire à l'angiographie carotidienne dans le diagnostic et la surveillance des accidents vasculaires cérébraux. 8e Symposium neuroradiol. Paris 1967.

HOWRY, D. H.: Techniques used in ultrasonic visualization of soft tissue structures of the body. IRE, Convention Record **9**, 75—88 (1955).

— BLISS, R. W.: Ultrasonic visualization of soft tissue structures of the body. J. Lab. clin. Med. **40**, 579—592 (1952).

— GORDON, D.: Ultrasonic tomography. In: Ultrasound as a diagnostic and surgical tool. Ed.: D. GORDON. Edinburgh-London: Livingstone 1964, pp. 103—123.

— STOTT, D. A., BLISS, R. W.: The ultrasonic visualization of carcinomas of the breast and other soft-tissue structures. Cancer **7**, 354—358 (1954).

HSIA, D., KONX, W. E., PAINE, R. S.: A case of phenylketonuria with borderline intelligence. Amer. J. Dis. Child. **94**, 33 (1957).

HUETER, T. F.: Messung der Ultraschallabsorption in tierischen Geweben und ihre Abhängigkeit von der Frequenz. Naturwissenschaften **35**, 285—287 (1948).

— Messung der Ultraschallabsorption im menschlichen Schädelknochen und ihre Abhängigkeit von der Frequenz. Naturwissenschaften **39**, 12—22 (1952).

— BOLT, R. H.: An ultrasonic method for outlining the cerebral ventricles. J. acoust. Soc. Amer. **23**, 160—167 (1951).

ICHIHARA, A.: Studies on diagnostic application of ultrasound. II. Echo-encephalography. Med. J. Hiroshima Univ. **14**, 129—140 (1966).

— MASAOKA, Y., OTANI, M.: Examination of bone echo in normal skull using simple stereotaxic apparatus. Japan. Med. Ultrasonics **2**, 43—45 (1964).

IIZUKA, J. H.: Physikalische Eigenschaften des Ultraschalls. Intern. Symposium Echo-Encephalographie. Erlangen 14./15. April 1967.

— Correlation between neuroradiological and echoencephalographical findings. 8e Symposium neuroradiol. Paris 1967.

INABA, Y., MARUTA, H., HATA, H.: A study of cerebral edema by ultrasound. Japan. Med. Ultrasonics 1, Proc. 3rd Meeting of Japan. Soc. of Ultrasonics in Medicine. Tokyo: Juntendo University 1963, p. 13—14.

INUGAMI, K., HACHIYA, SASAKI, H., HAYASHI, A., WAGAI, T., ISHIKAWA, I., YUKISHITA K.: Ultrasonic attenuation in epilepsy. Japan. Med. Ultrasonics **2**, 57—58 (1964).

ISHII, M.: An experimental study of stereotaxic destruction on the cat brain by intense focused ultrasound—The improvement of the apparatus for experiment. Nihon Geka Hokan **34**, 619—633 (1965).

ISHIKAWA, S.: Attenuation of ultrasound in brain tissue. Nihon Geka Hokan **33**, 923—940 (1964).

— NONAKA, H., YUKISHITA, K.: Ultrasonic attenuation in brain tissue (4th report). Japan. Med. Ultrasonics **2**, 60—61 (1964).

— YUKISHITA, K., SATO, K., ITO, K., WAGAI, T.: Ultrasonic attenuation in brain tissue (7th report). Japan. Med. Ultrasonics **3**, 48 (1965).

ITO, K.: The clinical application of ultrasonics to the localization of brain tumors. Arch. jap. Chir. **33**, 770—799 (1964).

— ABE, Y., KIKUCHI, S.: Diagnostic application of ultrasound in intracerebral hemorrhage (4th report). Japan. Med. Ultrasonics **2**, 49—52 (1964).

— IISHIKAWA, S., WAGAI, T., UCHIDA, R.: Ultrasono-tomography of brain (the 2nd report)—contact-sector-scanning-tomography. Japan. Med. Ultrasonics **3**, 30 (1965).

— NAJAMURA, K.: The effects of ultrasonic waves on the growth of young bones. Japan. Med. Ultrasonics 1, Proc. 3rd Meeting Japan. Soc. of Ultrasonics in Medicine. Tokyo: Juntendo University 1963, p. 1.

Ito, K., Nonaka, H., Ohara, Y., Tanaka, K.: Diagnosis of brain tumor by ultrasound through the dura mater. Japan. Med. Ultrasonics **3**, 52 (1965).

— Sugawara, K., Ohara, Y., Abe, Y., Kikuchi, S.: Ultrasonics in the diagnosis of head injury—"Hematoma echoes" as an aid in the diagnosis of subdural and epidural hematoma. Japan. Med. Ultrasonics **4**, 39 (1966).

— Tanaka, K., Abe, Y.: Ultrasound in the diagnosis of head injuries. Intern. Symposium Echo-Encephalographie. Erlangen 14./15. April 1967.

Iwata, K., Watanabe, S., Tomiyasu, M.: A diagnostic method of brain tumors in using A-scope. Japan. Med. Ultrasonics **2**, 45—47 (1964).

Jackson, F. E., Hussey, M., Relyea, D.: Utilization of pulsed sonic beams (echoencephalogram) for detection of fragments of bone indriven into the brain. Milit. Med. **130**, 1107 to 1109 (1965).

Jacobi, G.: Irrtumsmöglichkeiten im Echo-Encephalogramm bei Kindern mit hirnatrophischen Prozessen. Intern. Symposium Echo-Encephalographie. Erlangen 14./15. April 1967.

— Kazner, E., Wollensak, J.: Subdurale Ergüsse und Hämatome bei Säuglingen und Kindern. Betrachtungen zur Pathogenese, Klinik, Therapie und Prognose. Z. Kindheilk. **96**, 199—227 (1966).

— Schuch, P.: Echo-Encephalographie und ihre Ergebnisse bei Kindern. Pädiat. Prax. **5**, 433—443 (1966).

— — Echo-Encephalographie und ihre Ergebnisse bei Kindern. Chir. Praxis **11**, 363—373 (1967).

— Stephan, U.: Über die Anwendungsmöglichkeiten der Echoencephalographie bei Kindern. Mschr. Kinderheilk. **133**, 344—345 (1965).

Jacobi, J., Kamm, P., Schwarz, W.: Bedeutung der Ultraschallkardiographie in der Herzdiagnostik. Materia Medica Nordmark **14**, 251—257 (1962).

Jacobi, M.: Anwendungsmöglichkeiten und Ergebnisse der Echoencephalographie im Kindesalter. Inaug.-Diss. Erlangen 1966.

Jacobsen, H. H., Melchlor, J. C.: Radium therapy and nuclear medicine. Amer. J. Roentgenol. **101**, 188 (1967).

James, T. G., Turner, E. A.: Traumatic intracranial hematoma. Lancet **1951 II**, 45—50.

Jamsson, F., Sundmark, E.: Determination of the velocity of ultrasound in ocular tissues at different temperatures. Acta Ophthal. (Kbh.) **39**, 899—910 (1961).

Janz, D.: Die Epilepsien. Stuttgart: Thieme 1969.

Jefferson, A.: Some experience with echo-encephalography. J. Neurol. Psychiat. **22**, 83—84 (1959).

— Clinical experiences with echo-encephalography. Acta neurochir. (Wien) **10**, 392—409 (1962).

— Hill, A. I.: Echo-Encephalography. Progr. neurol. Surg. **1**, pp. 64—93. Basel-New York: Karger 1966.

— — The importance of the non-midline echoes in A-scan echoencephalography with a commentary on their relevance to the reliability of the method. Symposium Echo-Encephalographie. Erlangen 14./15. April 1967.

Jeppson, St.: Echo-encephalography. III. Further studies on the sources of the midline echo and a clinical evaluation. Acta chir. scand. **119**, 445—462 (1960).

— Echo-encephalography. IV. The midline echo; an evaluation of its usefulness for diagnosing intracranial expansivities and investigation into its sources. Acta chir. scand. Suppl. **272**, 1—151 (1961).

— Echo-encephalography V. A method for recording the intracranial pressure with the aid of the echoencephalographic technique. A preliminary report. Acta chir. scand. **128**, 218 to 224 (1964).

— The use of the M-echo in clinical echoencephalography. Acta neurol. scand. **41**, Suppl. 13, 7—12 (1965).

— A method for recording the intracranial pressure with the aid of the echo-encephalographic technique. Intern. Symposium Echo-Encephalographie. Erlangen 14./15. April 1967.

JERVIS, G. A.: Phenylpyruvic oligophrenia: Introductory study of 50 cases of mental deficiency associated with excretion of phenylpyruvic acid. Arch. Neurol. Psychiat. **38**, 944 (1937).

— Phenylpyruvic oligophrenia (Phenylketonuria). Ass. Res. nerv. Dis. Proc. **33**, 259 (1954).

— Phenylpyruvic oligophrenia (Phenylketonuria). In: Genetics and the Inheritance of Integrated Neurological and Psychiatriy Patterns. Res. Publ. Ass. nerv. ment. Dis. **33**, 259 (1954).

JOYNER, C. R., REID, J. M., BOND, J. P.: Reflected ultrasound in the assessment of mitral valve disease. Circulation **27**, 503—511 (1963).

KALBERMATTEN, J. A. DE: Die EEG-Veränderungen bei Stammganglien — resp. tiefsitzenden subkortikalen Großhirntumoren. Psychiat. et Neurol. (Basel) **139**, 249—284 (1960).

KANAYA, H., YAMASAKI, H., SAIKI, I.: Study of echoencephalography of intracerebral hematomas. Japan. Med. Ultrasonics **1**, 15—16 (1963).

KAISER, SILVIA, BICKEL, H.: Psychological and Developmental Evaluation of Phenylketonuric Patients Treated with a Phenylalanine-restricted Diet. Heidelberg Symposium on Phenylketonuria. Stuttgart: Thieme (in press).

KATANUMA, M., AZAMI, S., TSUTSUMI, Y.: Pen-writing echo-encephalograph. Japan. Med. Ultrasonics **2**, 52—54 (1964).

KAUTZKY, R., ZÜLCH, K. J.: Neurologisch-Neurochirurgische Röntgendiagnostik und andere Methoden zur Erkennung intrakranialer Erkrankungen. Berlin-Göttingen-Heidelberg: Springer 1955.

KAZNER, E.: Die Echoenzephalographie beim epiduralen Haematom. Acta neurochir. (Wien) **13**, 582 (1965).

— Erkennung und Differentialdiagnose intrakranieller Komplikationen nach Schädel-Hirn-Trauma. Intern. Symposium Echo-Encephalographie. Erlangen 14./15. April 1967.

— KUNZE, ST.: Echo-encephalographische Befunde bei Tumoren der Mittellinie und der Schädelbasis. Intern. Symposium Echo-Encephalographie. Erlangen 14./15. April 1967.

— — SCHIEFER, W.: Die Bedeutung der Echoencephalographie für die Erkennung epiduraler Haematome. Langenbecks Arch. klin. Chir. **310**, 267—291 (1965).

— — — Echoencephalography as an aid to the diagnosis of space-occupying lesions in the posterior fossa by measuring the size of the third and lateral ventricles. J. Neurosurg. **26**, 511—520 (1967).

— SCHIEFER, W.: Das Ultraschall-Echo-Verfahren (Echoencephalographie), eine Methode zur frühzeitigen Erkennung raumfordernder intrakranieller Prozesse. Med. Mschr. **18**, 27—31 (1964).

— — Operative Entfernung eines Zystizerkus aus dem IV. Ventrikel. Med. Bild-Dienst Roche, Heft 3, 18—23 (1965).

— — Echoencephalographische Untersuchungsergebnisse bei Schädel-Hirnverletzungen. Acta radiol. 5, diagnosis, 7th Symposium neuroradiol., New York 1964, 832—842 (1966).

— — Die Echoencephalographie bei raumfordernden Prozessen der hinteren Schädelgrube. Acta Neurochir. (Wien) **14**, 177—196 (1966).

— — The diagnosis of epidural haematoma on the basis of echo-encephalography. Excerpta medica, International Congress Series **139**, No. 173 (1967).

KEIDEL, W.-D.: Über die Verwendung des Ultraschalls in der klinischen Diagnostik. Ärztl. Forschg. Wörishofen **1**, 349—357 (1947).

KELLY, E.: Ultrasonic energy. Biological investigations and medical applications. Urbana: University of Illinois Press 1965.

KESSLER, G. B.: Echoencephalography. Its use as a diagnostic aid in neurological disease; plus a comparison with EEG foci. Bull. Los Angeles neurol. Soc. **30**, 21—26 (1965).

KIENAST, H. W., BOSHES, L.: Echoencephalographic studies in epilepsy. Proceedings 8th Intern. Congress Neurol. Vienna 5—10 Nov., 1965.

KIKUCHI, S., ITO, K.: Ultrasonic diagnosis of intracranial disease. Rinsho Geka (Clin. Surg., Tokyo) **18**, 376—381 (1963).

— — ABE, Y.: Diagnosis of apoplexy by ultrasonic pulses (2nd report). Japan. Med. Ultrasonics **2**, 53—56 (1963).

Kikuchi, S., Uchida, R., Tanaka, K., Wagai, T.: Early cancer diagnosis through ultrasonic. J. acoust. Soc. Amer. **29**, 824—833 (1957).

Kinney, W. M. Mc, Thurstone, F. L., Avant, W. S., Wallace, W. K.: The significance of intracerebral echo pulsations. In: Diagnostic Ultrasound. New York: Plenum Press 1966.

— Toole, J. J., Sharp, W. T., MacMillan, E. A., Gibson, J. W., South, B. D.: Evaluation of five hundred psychiatric in-patients by midline echoencephalography. Acta radiol. (Stockh.) **5**, 865—870 (1966).

Knox, W. E.: An evaluation of the treatment of phenylketonuria with diets low in phenylalanine. Pediatrics **26**, 1 (1960).

Koslowski, L., Thies, W.: Bericht über 5900 Schädel-Hirn-Traumen. Mschr. Unfallheilk. **67**, 97—103 (1964).

— — Erfahrungen mit der Echo-Encephalographie bei frischen Schädel-Hirn-Traumen. Unfallheilk. **97**, 170—172 (1966).

Kossoff, G., Robinson, D. E., Garrett, W. J.: Two dimensional ultrasonograph in obstetrics. In: Diagnostic Ultrasound. New York: Plenum Press 1966.

— — Liu, C. N., Garrett, W. J.: Design criteria for ultrasonic visualization system. Ultrasonics **2**, 29—38 (1964).

Kramer, G.: Zur Diagnostik raumfordernder intrakranieller Prozesse mit Hilfe des Echoimpulsverfahrens. Chirurg **34**, 290—298 (1963).

— Die Echoenzephalographie. Dtsch. med. Wschr. **89**, 564—567 (1964).

— Vierjährige Erfahrungen mit der Echoencephalographie bei Schädelhirntraumen. Mschr. Unfallheilk. **69**, 145—150 (1966).

— Schwierigkeiten in der Deutung echo-encephalographischer Befunde bei Schädelhirntraumen. Intern. Symposium Echo-Encephalographie. Erlangen 14./15. April 1967.

Kratochwil, A.: Die Bedeutung der Ultraschalldiagnostik für Geburtshilfe und Gynäkologie. Schweiz. med. Wschr. **99**, 992—997 (1969).

Krauland, W.: Über die Quellen des akuten und chronischen subduralen Hämatoms. Stuttgart: Thieme 1961.

Krautkrämer, J., Krautkrämer, H.: Werkstoffprüfung mit Ultraschall. Berlin-Heidelberg-New York: Springer 1966.

Kresse, H.: Über die physikalischen Gesetzmäßigkeiten bei Anwendung des Ultraschall-Echoverfahrens am Schädel. Intern. Symposium Echo-Encephalographie. Erlangen 14./15. April 1967.

Kroll, W., Mostafawy, A.: Caudales Hypoplasiesyndrom mit zusätzlichen Mißbildungen bei unbalancierter Translokation. Z. Kinderheilk. **107**, 246—251, 13—15 (1969).

Kruse, R.: Das myklonisch-astatische Petit Mal. Berlin-Heidelberg-New York: Springer 1968.

Kugler, J.: Elektroencephalographie in Klinik und Praxis. Stuttgart: Thieme 1963.

Kunze, St.: Die operative Behandlung intracerebraler Blutungen unter besonderer Berücksichtigung des Spontanhämatoms. Inauguraldissertation, Erlangen 1964.

— Inwieweit kann die Echo-Encephalographie zur Differentialdiagnose Hirnblutung-Erweichung beitragen? Intern. Symposium Echo-Encephalographie. Erlangen 14./15. April 1967.

Kurze, Th., Dyck, O., Barrows, H. S.: Neurosurgical evaluation of ultrasonic encephalograph. J. Neurosurg. **22**, 437—440 (1965).

L'Ahoda, F., Neundörfer, B.: Übersichten Ultraschallechoencephalographie. Klin. Wschr. **61 a**, 46. Jg., Heft 16, 849—856 (1968).

Lang, K.: Die phenylpyruvische Oligophrenie. Ergebn. inn. Med. Kinderheilk. **6**, 78 (1955).

Lang, W., Pia, H. W.: Prognose und Indikation zur Ventrikulocisternostomie (Torkildsen-Operation). Dtsch. Z. Nervenheilk. **182**, 176—184 (1961).

Langevin, M. P.: Les ondes ultrasonores. Rev. gén. électr. **23**, 626—634 (1928).

Lapayowker, M. S., Christen, G. E.: Echoencephalography in general hospital practice. Amer. J. Roentgenol. **93**, 803—810 (1965).

— Murtagh, F., Kirkpatrick, J. A.: Echoencephalography in the evaluation of hydrocephalus. Radiology **86**, 1052—1055 (1966).

Lauber, H.: Das Pneumencephalogramm. Meßverfahren bei Erwachsenen. München: Joh. Ambrosius Barth 1965.

LAUSBERG, G., GELETNEKY, C. L.: Frühdiagnose, Therapie und Verlaufsformen des Hydrocephalus bei cystischen Dysrhaphien. Zbl. Neurochir. **28**, 161—168 (1967).

— — Aspekte zum Hydrocephalus bei cystischen Dysrhaphien. Z. Kinderheilk. **105**, 147 bis 155 (1969).

LEE, R. G., MORLEY, T.: The routine use of echoencephalography in the diagnosis of intracranial masses. Canad. med. Ass. J. **91**, 987—990 (1964).

LEHMANN, J. ST., EVANS, G. C., BRADY, L. W.: Ultrasound exploration of the spleen. In: Diagnostic Ultrasound. New York: Plenum Press 1966.

LEKSELL, L.: Behandling av akuta skallskador och deras följdtillstånd. Kirurgisk behandling. Nord. Med. **54**, 1444 (1955).

— Kirurgisk behandling av skallskador. Vortrag Meeting of Svenska läkarsällskapet. Stockholm 7. Dec. 1954.

— Echo-Encephalography. I. Detection of intracranial complications following head injury. Acta chir. scand. **110**, 301—315 (1955/56).

— Echo-Encephalography. II. Midline echo from the pineal body as an index of pineal displacement. Acta chir. scand. **115**, 225—259 (1958).

LE MAY, M. J., OJEMANN, R. G.: Angiography changes associated with a dilated temporal horn. Acta radiol. (Stockh.), Diagnosis **1**, 358—366 (1963).

LEPINTRE, J., LEFEBVRE, J., DEBRUNI, G., LEGAL, J.: Transillumination et échoencéphalographie. Examens physiques simples dans diagnostic et dans la surveillance des collections liquidiennes sousdurales chez l'enfant. Neurochirurgie **11**, 285—293 (1963).

LEPOIRE, J., LAPRAS, CL.: L'échoventriculographie. Neurochirurgie **13**, 256—258 (1967).

LHOTSKY, J., WEISS, F.: Erfahrungen mit der Echo-Encephalographie am chirurgischen Krankengut. Intern. Symposium Echo-Encephalographie. Erlangen 14./15. April 1967.

LITHANDER, B.: A control method for echo-encephalography. Acta psychiat. scand. **35**, 235 to 240 (1960).

— The clinical use of echo-encephalography. Acta psychiat. scand. **35**, 241—244 (1960).

— Origin of echoes in the echo-encephalogram. J. Neurol. Psychiat. **24**, 22—31 (1961).

— Clinical and experimental studies in echo-encephalography. Acta psychiat. scand. **36**, Suppl. 159 (1961).

— The true displacement of the midline brain structures in relation to midline echo displacement. Acta psychiat. scand. **36**, Suppl. 159, 9—12 (1961).

— Estimation of the experimental error and normal individual variation in echo-encephalography and other methods of diagnosing extracerebral haematomas. Acta psychiat. scand. **36**, Suppl. 159, 31—36 (1961).

— Echo-encephalography in children. Acta psychiat. scand. **36**, Suppl. 159, 37—50 (1961).

— Echoencephalography. In: Technical Progress in Neurolgical Dialnostics. Ed.: O. GIL-

— Echo-encephalography and extracerebral haematomas. Comparison between echoencephalography in children. Acta psychiat. scand. **36**, Suppl. 159, 37—50 (1961).

— Echoencephalography. A general survey. Acta neurol. scand. **41**, Suppl. 13, 1—6 (1965).

— Echoencephalography. In: Technical Progress in Neurological Diagnostics. Hrsg.: O. GILLAND. Amsterdam: Elsevier 1965.

— MARIONS, O.: Echo-encephalography in adults. Acta psychiat. scand. **36**, Suppl. 159, 18 to 30 (1961).

LOMBROSO, C. I., ERBA, G.: The use and limitations of two-dimensional echoencephalography. Intern. Symposium Echo-Encephalographie. Erlangen 14./15. April 1967.

— — YOGO, T.: Two-dimensional ultrasonography: A method to study normal and abnormal ventricles. Pediatrics **42**, 157—174 (1968).

LÖPPING, B.: Klinische und experimentelle Ultraschalluntersuchungen bei Augen mit Netzhautablösung und intraokularen Tumoren. Inaugural-Diss. Köln 1962.

LOW, N. L., BOSMA, J. F., ARMSTRONG, M. D.: Studies of phenylketonuria. VI. EEG studies in phenylketonuria. Arch. Neurol. Psychiat. (Chic.) **77**, 359 (1957).

LUDWIG, G. D.: The velocity of sound through tissues and the acoustic impedance of tissues. J. acoust. Soc. Amer. **22**, 862—866 (1950).

— BOLT, R. H., HUETER, T. F., BALLANTINE, H. T.: Factors influencing the use of ultrasounds as a diagnostic aid. Trans. Amer. neurol. Ass. **75**, 225—228 (1950).

LYNN, J. G., PUTNAM, T. J.: Histology of cerebral lesions produced by focused ultrasound. Amer. J. Path. **20**, 637—649 (1944).

MAGNUS, O., STORM VAN LEEUWEN, W., COBB, W. A. (Ed.): Electroencephalography and cerebral tumors. Electroenceph. clin. Neurophysiol. Suppl. **19**, 1961.

MAKOW, D. M.: Délimitation des contours ventriculaires par les ultrasons. Neurochirurgie **10**, 467—469 (1964).

— MCRAE, D. L.: Echo-Tomographie des Schädels. Image Roche, Heft 4, 1966, S. 15—22.

— — Horizontal scanning of the head with ultrasound. Med. biol. Engng. **5**, 33—40 (1967).

— — Two-dimensional echoencephalography: recent results. Intern. Symposium Echo-Encecephalhgraphie. Erlangen 14./15. April 1967.

— REAL, R. R.: Development of a 360° compound immersion head scanner. In: Diagnostic ultrasound. Eds.: C. C. GROSSMAN et al. New York: Plenum Press 1966, pp. 166—185.

— WYSLOUZIL, W., WHITE, D. N., BLANCHARD, J.: Novel immersion scanner and display system for ultrasonic brain tomography. Acta radiol. 5, diagnosis, 7th Symposium neuroradiol., New York 1964, 855—864 (1966).

MALAMUD, N.: Neuropathology of phenylketunuria. J. Neuropath. exp. Neurol. **25**, 154 (1966).

MALECI, O.: L'elettroencefalografia nei tumori cerebrali. Padova: Cedam 1952.

MARUTA, H., HATA, H., YAMAOKA, K., INABA, Y.: A study of the ultrasonic attenuation of the brain during anaesthesia—The ultrasonic monitoring of anaesthesia. Japan. Med. Ultrasonics **2**, 54—57 (1964).

MATAUSCHEK, J.: Einführung in die Ultraschalltechnik. Berlin: Verlag Technik 1957.

MATSON, D. D.: Cerebellar astrocytoma in childhood. Pediatrics **18**, 150—158 (1956).

MATTHES, K., RECH, W.: Der Ultraschall in der Medizin. Kongreßbericht der Erlanger Ultraschall-Tagung 1949. Zürich: Hirzel 1949.

MAUTNER, H., QUINN, K. V.: Phenylpyruvic oligophrenia. Ann. paediat. **172**, 1 (1949).

MCGINNIS, K. D., ZYLAK, C. J.: Echoencephalography as an adjuvant to the routine examination of the skull. Radiology **85**, 291—297 (1965).

MCKINNEY, W. M.: The value of R-mode determination of midline echo in echoencephalography. Neurology (Minneap.) **14**, 259 (1964).

— AVANT, W. S., THURSTONE, F. L., BETTE POU: Intracranial pulsations as measured by ultrasound. Engin. Med. Biol. Proc. of the 18th Ann. Conf. 1965, p. 68,

— THURSTONE, F. L., AVANT, W. S., WALLACE, W. K.: The significance of intracranial echo pulsations. In: Diagnostic ultrasound. Eds.: C. C. GROSSMAN et al. New York: Plenum Press 1966, pp. 114—116.

— TOOLE, J. F., SHARP, W. T., MCMILLAN, E. A., GIBSON, J. W., SOUTH, B. B.: Evaluation of five hundred psychiatric inpatients by midline echoencephalography. Acta radiol. 5, diagnosis, 7th Symposium neuroradiol., New York 1964, 865—870 (1966).

MCLAURIN. R. L., HELMER, F.: Angiographic observations following removal of subdural hematomas. Acta radiol. 5, diagnosis, 7th Symposium neuroradiol., New York 1964, 381 to 387 (1966).

MCRAE, D. L., MAKOW, D. M.: Horizontal laminography of the head with ultrasound. Further results. 8e Syomposium neuroradiol. Paris 1967.

METZEL, E., UMBACH, W.: Akute posttraumatische Blutungen des Schädelinneren. Actuelle Chir. **1**, 145—152 (1966).

MICSKY, L. I. VON: Ultrasonic tomography in obstetrics and gynecology. In: Diagnostic Ultrasound. New York: Plenum Press 1966.

MIKKELSEN, B.: Ekkoencefalografie. Nord. Med. **77**, 347—352 (1967).

MIKOL, F.: L'écho-encéphalographie. Presse méd. **73**, 729—730 (1965).

MILBLED, G., WIREMBLEWSKI, F., RAMEZ, T.: L'écho-encéphalographie. Exploration cérébrale par les ultrasons. Lille méd. **9**, 712—715 (1964).

MILLICHAP, J. G., BICKFORD, R. G., MILLER, R. H., BACKUS, R. E.: The electroencephalogram in children with intracranial tumors and seizures. Neurology **12**, 329—336 (1962).

MILLNER, R., RICHWIEN, R.: Grundlagen der medizinischen Elektronik. Frankfurt a. M.: Akademische Verlagsgesellschaft 1969.

MITSUNO, T., KANAYA, H., SHIRAKATA, S., ASHAWA, K., ISHIKAWA, Y.: Surgical treatment of hypertensive intracerebral hemorrhage. J. Neurosurg. **24**, 70—76 (1966).

Mizuno, Sh., Takeuchi, H., Nakano, K.: Diagnostic application of ultrasound in obstetrics and gynecology. In: Diagnostic Ultrasound. New York: Plenum Press 1966.

Mostafawy, A., Czettritz v. G., Kruse, R.: Echoencephalographische Seitenventrikelmessung bei Kindern. 1. Weltkongreß Ultraschalldiagnostik der Medizin. Wien 1969.

— Nagle, J., Newill, A., Braatz, E.: A study of cerebral atrophy in phenylketonuria. A sonoencephalographic examination of 45 PKU patients. Neuropädiatrie **2**, 215—225 (1970).

— — The combined electroencephalographic and sonoencephalographic examination (in press).

Mühlhäuser, O.: Verfahren zur Zustandsbestimmung von Werkstoffen, besonders zur Ermittlung von Fehlern darin. DRP 569 598 (1931).

Müller, H. R.: Zur Echoencephalographie; ihre Indikation beim Schädel-Hirntrauma. Schweiz. med. Wschr. **94**, 119—124 (1964).

— Diagnose des epiduralen Hämatoms im präklinischen Stadium. Zum Wert der routinemäßigen Echoencephalographie bei Schädelkalottenfrakturen. Schweiz. med. Wschr. **97**, 1055—1057 (1967).

— Klingler, M.: Problematik der postoperativen Echolotung. Intern. Symposium Echo-Encephalographie. Erlangen 14./15,. April 1967.

Mumenthaler, M.: Neurologie für Ärzte und Studenten. Stuttgart: Thieme 1969.

Mundt, G. H., Jr., Hughes, W. F., Jr.: Ultrasonics in ocular diagnosis. Amer. J. Ophthal. **41**, 488—498 (1956).

Nadjmi, M.: Beziehungen zwischen Röntgen-Anatomie und Echo-Encephalographie. Intern. Symposium Echo-Encephalographie. Erlangen 14./15. April 1967.

Nagai, H., Sakurai, K., Hayashi, M., Furuse, M., Okamura, K.: Echoencephalogram following experimental intracerebral hemorrhage and infarction. Proc. 3rd Meeting Japan. Soc. Ultrasonics in Medicine. Tokyo: Juntendo University 1963, p. 15.

— — — — — Shintani, A., Kobayashi, T.: Ultrasonic findings in intracranial diseases—Analyis of 114 cases. Japan. Med. Ultrasonics **2**, 47—49 (1964).

Newell, J. A.: The use of ultrasonics in medical diagnosis. Proc. 3rd Int. Conf. Med. Electron. London: Institution of Electrical Engineers 422—424 (1961).

— Ultrasonic localization. Brit. J. Radiol. **34**, 546—550 (1961).

— Ultrasonics in medicine. Phys. in Med. Biol. **8**, 241—264 (1963).

Nichols, R. A., Whisnant, J. P., Baker, H. L., Jr.: A-mode echoencephalography: Its value and limitations and report of 200 verified cases. Mayo Clin. Proc. **43**, 36—53 (1968).

Nicholson, A. M.: Piezo-electric effect in composite Rochelle salt crystal. Proc. Amer. Inst. Elect. Eng. **38**, 1467—1493 (1919).

Nonaka, H., Yukishita, K., Ishikawa, S., Ito, K.: Experimental brain edema by ultrasound. Japan. Med. Ultrasonics **2**, 9—11 (1964).

Nover, A.: Klinische Ultraschalluntersuchungen bei Netzhautablösung und intraokularen Tumoren. Klin. Mbl. Augenheilk. **142**, 168—186 (1963).

— Stallkamp, H.: Experimentelle Ultraschalluntersuchungen bei Augen mit intraokularen Fremdkörpern. Albrecht v. Graefes Arch. Ophthal. **164**, 517—523 (1962).

— — Über die Möglichkeiten und Grenzen der Ultraschalldiagnostik intraokularer Fremdkörper. Bericht über die Zusammenkunft d. Deutsch. Ophthalm. Ges., Heidelberg 1960. München: Bergmann 1960, S. 251—255.

Nürnberger, S., Schaltenbrand, G.: Messungen am Encephalogramm. Ein Beitrag zum Begriff des „normalen Encephalogramms". Dtsch. Z. Nervenheilk. **174**, 1—14 (1955).

Oberschulte-Beckmann, D., Otto, D.: Das anatomische Substrat des Endechos in der Echo-Encephalographie aus der Sicht des Experiments. Intern. Symposium Echo-Encephalographie. Erlangen 14./15. April 1967.

— — Echo-encephalische Untersuchungen an Leichenschädeln mit künstlichen epiduralen Hämatomen. Intern. Symposium Echo-Encephalographie. Erlangen 14./15. April 1967.

— — Nachweis künstlicher epiduraler Hämatome durch Echo-Encephalographie. Erlangen 14./15. April 1967.

— — Nachweis künstlicher epiduraler Hämatome durch Echo-Encephalographie. Chirurg **38**, 370—373 (1967).

Odom, G. L., Davis, C. H., Woodhall, B.: Brain tumors in children. Clinical analysis of 164 cases. Pediatrics **18**, 856—870 (1956).

Ohara, Y., Abe, Y., Ishikawa, S., Ito, K., Tanaka, K.: Ultrasonotomography of brain (3rd report). Med. Ultrasonics **4**, 61 (1966).

Oka, M.: Experiences of cranial test by measuring the ultrasonic loss in traumatic brain. Proc. 3rd Meeting Japan. Soc. of Ultrasonics in Medicine. Tokyo: Juntendo University 1963, p. 14.

— Natto, Y., Sakamoto, H., Kijiraoka, Y., Kiyoshima, K.: Study on the dynamic test of head injury by measuring the ultrasonic attenuation of traumatized brains—The ultrasonic attenuation of injured brains. Japan. Med. Ultrasonics **2**, 58—60 (1964).

Oksala, A., Lehtinen, A.: Über die diagnostische Verwendung von Ultraschall in der Augenheilkunde. Ophthalmologica **134**, 387—395 (1957).

— — Diagnosis of detachment of the retina by means of ultrasound. Acta opthal. **35**, 461 to 467 (1957).

— — Das Echogramm in der Diagnostik von Augenkrankheiten. Klin. Mbl. Augenheilk. **137**, 72—87 (1960).

— — Experimental observations on acoustic biomicroscopy of various parts of the eye. Acta ophthal. **38**, 599—605 (1960).

— — Acoustic biomicroscopy of intraocular tumors. Amer. J. Ophthal. **51**, 1203—1211 (1961).

Oldendorf, W. H.: Ultrasound in neurologic diagnosis. Trans. Bio-Med. Engin. B. M. E. **II**, 118—122 (1964).

Oldenkott, P.: Echoencephalographie. Kritisches zu einer Untersuchungsmethode. Med. Welt **44**, 2427—2429 (1968).

Ossoinig, K.: Ultrasonic diagnosis on the eye—an aid for the clinic (review). In: Ultrasonics in Ophthalmology. Münster: Symposium 1966, S. 116—133.

Overton, M. C., Coe, J. E., Snodgrass, S. R.: Echoencephalography: a clinical appraisal. Tex. St. J. Med. **61**, 823—829 (1965).

P'an, Y.-H., Wu, H.-H., Ch'en, K.-P., Su, M.-F.: Ultrasonics in the diagnosis of intracranial space-occupying lesions. Zhong. Waike Z. (Peking) **11**, 536—541 (1963).

Paine, R. S.: The variability in manifestation of untreated patients with phenoylketonuria. Pediatrics **20**, 290 (1957).

Pantschenko, D. I., Matscheret, E. L.: Unsere Erfahrungen mit der Echo-Encephalographie. Intern. Symposium Echo-Encephalographie. Erlangen 14./15. April 1967.

Parkinson, D., Chochinov, H.: Subdural hematomas—some observations on their postoperative course. J. Neurosurg. **17**, 901—904 (1960).

Pell, R. L.: Ultrasound for routine clinical investigations. Ultrasonics **2**, 87—89 (1964).

Penzholz, H.: Zur Diagnose traumatischer intrakranieller Blutungen unter besonderer Berücksichtigung von Carotisangiographie und Echoencephalographie. Forschung, Praxis, Fortbildung **11**, 390—397 (1966).

Pepin, B., Jaquinot, B., Gendelin, B.: L'écho-encéphalographie. Méd. int. **1**, 35—40 (1966).

Perry, T. L., Hansen, S., Tischler, B., Bunting, R., Diamond, S.: Glutamine depletion in phenylketonuria: possible cause of mental defect. New Engl. J. Med. **282**, 761 (1970).

Persson, A., Wennberg, A., Widen, L.: Experiences with echoencephalography in combination with EEG. Elektroenceph. clin. Neurophysiol. Suppl. **25** (1967).

Peters, G.: Ultraschallwirkung auf das Nervensystem. Kongreßbericht der Erlanger Ultraschalltagung. Zürich: Hirzel 1949, p. 166.

— Morpohologische Untersuchungen über die Wirkung von Ultraschallwellen auf das Zentralnervensystem. Fortschr. Neurol. Psychiat. **17**, 85—94 (1949).

— Die Wirkung der Ultraschallwellen auf das Zentralnervensystem. Strahlentherapie **79**, 643—658 (1949).

— Experimentelle Ultraschallschäden am Gehirn. Utraschall in Med. **4**, 60—62 (1952).

— Schädigung des Zentralnervensystems durch Ultraschall. In: Handb. spez. path. Anatomie u. Histologie, III. Teil. Berlin: Springer 1955.

Peyton, W.: First clinical use of ultrasound in localization of brain tumors in operating room. Zit. nach J. J. Wild and J. M. Reid (1953).

PIA, H. W.: Stellung und Entwicklung der Neurochirurgie in der Bundesrepublik und in Hessen. Memorandum an die Hessische Staatsregierung 1964.

PIA, H. W.: Zur Frage der Umgehungsdrainage nach Torkildsen. Zbl. Neurochir. **13**, 103—107 (1953).

— Hirnverletzungen bei Kindern und ihre akuten Komplikationen. Münch. med. Wschr. **108**, 760—768 (1966).

— Die Echoenzephalographie in der Hirngeschwulstdiagnostik. Dtsch. med. Wschr. **92**, 999 bis 1002 (1967).

— GELETNEKY, C. L.: Echo-Encephalographie bei infantilen Encephalopathien und ihren Folgen. Intern. Symposium Echo-Encephalographie. Erlangen 14./15. April 1967.

— — Echoenzephalographie. Thieme: Stuttgart 1968.

PLANTOL, TH.: La gamma-encéphalographie dans le diagnostic des lésions expansives intracrâniennes. Confin. neurol. (Basel) **21**, 137—158 (1961).

— L'écho-éncephalographie dans la détection des néoformations intracrâniennes. Neurochirurgie **13**, 19—22 (1967).

— Résultats de quatre années d'écho-encéphalographie dans les tumeurs cérébrales. Intern. Symposium Echo-Encephalographie. Erlangen 14./15. April 1967.

— Enregistrement d'écho-pulsations cérébrales et comparaison avec les oscillations rheoencéphalographiques. Intern. Symposium Echo-Encephalographie. Erlangen 14./15. April 1967.

— BETTI, O.: Diagnostic des méningiomes intracrâniens par la gamma-encéphalographie. Rev. neurol. **105**, 420—429 (1961).

— FISCHGOLD, H., DAVID, M., SACHS, M., COURSON, B.: Sur les examens physiques ambulatoires du cerveau. Intérêt de l'écho-encéphalographie médiane dans une observation d'emphysème sousdural. Neurochirurgie **11**, 274—284 (1965).

— METZGER, J., DAVID, M., FISCHGOLD, H.: Explorations techniques ambulatoires dans le diagnostic des tumeurs cérébrales hémispheriques. Acta radiol. 5, diagnosis, 7th Symposium neuroradiol., New York 1964, 906—914 (1966).

— MIKOL, F., CHARPENTIER, J., BUISSON, J.: L'écho-encéphalographie. Premiers résultats après six mois d'investigation en neurochirurgie. Rev. neurol. **110**, 489—505 (1964).

POHLMANN, R.: Die Ultraschalltherapie. Bern: Huber 1951.

— Über die Möglichkeit einer akustischen Abbildung in Analogie zur optischen. Z. Phys. (Berlin) **113**, 967—709 (1939).

— Die Ultraschalltherapie. Praktische Anwendung des Ultraschalls in der Medizin. Berlin: Huber 1951.

— Die neuesten Ergebnisse der Ultraschallforschung und Ausblick auf die moderne Technik. Arbeitsgemeinschaft für Forschung des Landes Nordrhein-Westfalen 101 (1961). 7—46 Westdeutscher Verlag Köln.

— Über die erforderlichen Voraussetzungen einer brauchbaren Ultraschall-Diagnostik. Rehabilitation **15**, 135 (1962).

— Über die Absorption des Ultraschalls im menschlichen Gewebe und ihre Abhängigkeit von der Frequenz. Phys. Z. (Berlin) **40**, 159—161 (1939).

— Über die erforderlichen Voraussetzungen einer brauchbaren Ultraschall-Diagnostik. Physikal. Med. **15**, 135 (1962) i. Tagungsber. Wiss. Vereinig. US-Forschung 1962.

PORRAS, C. L.: La ecoencefalografia en del diagnostico de los procesos intracraneales. Rev. clin. esp. **89**, 29—32 (1963).

POSER, C. M., VAN BOGAERT, L.: Neuropathological observations in PKU. Brain **82**, 1 (1959).

POZO, L. DEL, ANASTASIO Y ALIJARDE, J. V.: Ecos ventriculares en la exploración ultrasónica cerebral. Rev. clin. esp. **100**, 48—49 (1966).

PRIDIE, R. B., BROODIE, V.: The shift of the mid-line demonstrated ultrasonically in cerebral atrophy. 8e Symposium neuroradiol. Paris 1967.

PROLER, M. L., NORTH, R. R., LOW, M. D.: Echoencephalography—The measurement of the position of the midline structures in the skull by pulsed ultrasound. Med. Rec. (Houston) **57**, 416—417 (1964).

RADDA, H., SCHIMA, E.: Wert und Grenzen der Echoencephalographie bei frischen Schädel-Hirnverletzungen. Wien. med. Wschr. **115**, 881—883 (1965).

RASKIND, R.: Clinical studies in echoencephalography. Preliminary report. J. int. Coll. Surg. 42, 512—515 (1964).
RASKIND, R.: Clinical studies in echoencephalography: Report of 600 scans. J. int. Coll. Surg. 44, 153—158 (1965).
— Diagnostic ultrasonography. J. Amer. Geriat. Soc. 13, 887—892 (1965).
REID, J.: A review of some basic limitations in ultrasonic diagnosis. In: Proc. intern. Conf. Diag. Ultrasound, Pittsburgh 1965. New York: Plenum Press 1966, pp. 1—12.
REID, J. M., WILD, J. J.: Ultrasonic ranging for cancer diagnosis. Electronics (N. Y.), July 1952.
— — Ultrasonic echo-ranging for tissue diagnostic studies. IRE, Convention Record 9, 68 to 74 (1955).
REIHER, J., SANDOK, B. A., KLASS, D. W., WHISNANT, J. P.: Combined electroencephalography-sonoencephalography in temporal lobe epilepsy. Neurology (Minneap). (In press.)
RICHARDSON, A.: The management of primary intracranial hemorrhage. Modern trends in in neurology (third series). London: Butterworth & Co. 1962, pp. 89—107.
— AMBROSE, J.: Echoencephalography in cerebral hemorrhage and infarction. Lancet 1966 I, 319.
RICHARDSON, E. G.: Ultrasonic physics. Sec. Ed. Amsterdam: Elsevier Publ. Co. 1962.
RICHTER, H., KOSLOWSKI, L., LAU, G.: Der Wert der Echo-Encephalographie bei den akutlebensbedrohlichen, gedeckten Schädel-Hirnverletzungen. Intern. Symposium Echo-Encephalographie. Erlangen 14./15. April 1967.
ROBERTSON, E. G.: Pneumencephalography. Springfield (Ill.): Thomas 1957.
ROBINSON, D. E., KOSSOFF, G.: The C. A. L. two channel echo-encephaloscope. Ultrasonics 3, 69—74 (1965).
RUSSO, G. L., ARNOLD, J. G.: Neurosurgical experience with echoencephalography. W. Ann. D. C. 33, 260—264 (1964).
SAIER, J., PAILLAS, J., VIGOUROUX, R., GASTAUT, H.: Intérêt de l'échoencéphalographie pour le diagnostic neuro-chirurgical. Rev. neurol. 111, 520—522 (1964).
SANDEN, K. v.: Schalleistungsmessung in der Therapie und die Grenzen ihrer dosimetrischen Anwendbarkeit. Ultraschall in Med. I, 45—52 (1949).
SANDOK, B. A., REIHER, J., WHISNANT, J. P.: Combined electroencephalography and sonoencephalography. Mayo clin. Proc. 43, 628—634 (1968).
SCHÁB, R., KOPA, J.: Az echoencephalographiáról (Über die Echoencephlaographie). Orv. Hetil. 106, 1745—1752 (1965).
SCHEID, W.: Lehrbuch der Neurologie. Stuttgart: Thieme 1963.
SCHERZER, E.: Die Echoenzephalographie als Ergänzung des EEGs und ihre Grenzen. Wien. med. Wschr. 115, 957—959 (1965).
— Das normale Echoenzephalogramm und seine Bedeutung in der Traumatologie. Wien. klin. Wschr. 78, 301—304 (1966).
SCHIEFER, W.: Verbesserte Indikationsstellung zur Kontrastmitteluntersuchung durch vorhergehende Echoencephalographie. Dtsch. Röntgenkongreß 1964. Stuttgart: Thieme 1965, S. 326—330.
— Echo-Enzephalographie. Acta neurochir. (Wien) 13, 576—578 (1965).
— Raumbeschränkende Prozesse im Schädelinnern. Therapiewoche 16, 1471—1478 (1966).
— Die Echo-Encephalographie bei Tumoren im Bereich der Großhirnhemisphären. Intern. Symposium Echo-Encephalographie. Erlangen 14./15. April 1967.
— Zuverlässigkeit und Grenzen der eindimensionalen Echo-Encephalographie. Intern. Symposium Echo-Encephalographie. Erlangen 14./15. April 1967.
— Erkennung und Behandlung der traumatischen intrakraniellen Hämatome. Z. Schr. Therapiewoche 17, 38, 908 (1967).
— Fehler und Gefahren bei Kontrastmitteluntersuchungen im Kindesalter. Fortschr. Med. 85. Jg., Nr. 18 (1967).
— KAZNER, E.: Die Echo-Enzephalographie. Dtsch. med. Wschr. 89, 1394—1400 (1964).
— — Methodik und diagnostische Möglichkeiten der Echoencephalographie. Fortschr. Med. 84, 151—164 (1966).
— — Der heutige Stand der Echoencephalographie. Beitr. Neurochir. 13, 93—108 (1966).

Schiefer, W., Kazner, E., Brückner, H.: The diagnostic possibilities offered by echoencephalography. Excerpta medica, International Congress Series **60**, No. 58 (1963).
— — — Die Echoencephalographie, ihre Anwendungsweise und klinischen Ergebnisse. Fortschr. Neurol. Psychiat. **31**, 457—491 (1963).
— — Kunze, St.: Ergebnisse der Echoencephalographie bei supratentoriellen Geschwülsten. Zbl. Neurochir. **26**, 281—295 (1965).
— — — Clinical Echoencephalography. Berlin-Heidelberg-New York: Springer 1968.
— — — Möglichkeiten und Grenzen der Echoencephalographie beim Schädel-Hirntrauma. Dtsch. Ärztebl. **63**, 2645—2648, 2719—2722, 2777—2780, 2793—2794 (1966).
Schiersmann, O.: Einführung in die Enzephalographie. Leipzig: Thieme 1942.
Schiffer, K. H.: Zur Auswertung von Ventrikelbildern am Encephalogramm. Fortschr. Röntgenstr. **75**, 50—54 (1951).
Schlegel, J. U., Diggdon, P., Cueller, J.: The use of ultrasound for localizing renal calculi. J. Urol. **86**, 367 (1961).
Schmieder, F.: Das Encephalogramm nach Fleckfieber. Klin. Wschr. **26**, 14—19 (1948).
Schmitt, W., Braun, H.: Mitteilung der mittels Ultraschall-Kardiographie gewonnenen Ergebnisse bei Mitralvitien und Herzgesunden. Z. Kreisl.-Forsch. **49**, 214—222 (1960).
Scholz, W.: Contribution à l'anatomie pathologique du système nerveux central dans l'oligophrénie phénilpyruvique. L'Encéphale **46**, 668 (1957).
Schwan, H. P., Carstensen, E. L.: Advantages and limitations of ultrasonics in medicine. J. Amer. med. Ass. **149**, 121—125 (1952).
Segal, B. L., Likoff, W., Asperger, Z., Kingsley, B.: Ultrasound diagnosis of an abdominal aortic aneurysm. Amer. J. Cardiol. **17**, 101 (1966).
— — Kingsley, B.: Echocardiography; clinical application in mitralstenosis. J. Amer. med. Ass. **195**, 161 (1966).
Simon, Mikol, Hazemann: Zit. nach H. Fischgold: Die Schädelunfall-Diagnostik. Dtsch. Röntgenkongreß 1965. Stuttgart: Thieme 1966, S. 126—130.
Sjögren, I.: Echoencephalographic measurements of ventricular size in children. Develop. Med. Child. Neurol. **10**, 145—158 (1968).
— Echo-encephalography in infantile hydrocephalus. Acta paediat. scand. Suppl. **159**, 174 (1965).
— Echo-ventriculography in infantile hydrocephalus—preliminary report. Acta neurol. scand. **41**, Suppl. 13, 13—18 (1965).
— Echo-ventriculography in infantile hydrocephalus. In: Technical Progress in Neurological Diagnostics. Ed.: O. Gilland. Amsterdam: Elsevier 1965.
— Comparative studies between echoencephalography and cerebral pneumography in infantile hydrocephalus and cerebral malformations. Intern. Symposium Echo-Encephalographie. Erlangen 14./15. April 1967.
Skudrzyk, E.: Die physikalischen Ursachen für die mechanisch-chemisch-biologische Wirkung des Ultraschalls. Ultraschall in Med. **5**, 51—64 (1952).
Smyth, M.: Echoencephalographic technique. Philadelphia: Smith Kline-Precision Company 1963.
— Echoencephalography: Supplementary information on importance of far-side group of echoes. Ekoline Bulletin No. 3. Philadelphia: Smith-Kline-Precision Company 1964.
Sokoloff, S. J.: Ultraschallwellenmethoden zur Bestimmung innerer Defekte in Metallgegenständen. Zit. nach L. Bergmann.
Sokolow, S. J.: Zur Frage der Fortpflanzung ultraakustischer Schwingungen in verschiedenen Körpern. Elektr. Nachr. Techn. **6**, 454—461 (1929).
Somer, J. C.: Instantaneous and continuous pictures obtained by a new two-dimensional scan technique with a stationary transducer. Intern. Symposium Echo-Encephalographie. Erlangen 14./15. April 1967.
Stadler, V. H.: The EEG in phenylketonuria. Ann. Paediat. (Basel) **197**, 429 (1961).
Stallkamp, H.: Klinische und experimentelle Ultraschalluntersuchungen am gesunden Auge und bei intraokularen Fremdkörpern. Inaugural-Diss. Köln 1961.
— Nover, A.: Diagnostische Ultraschalluntersuchungen am gesunden Auge. Albrecht v. Graefes Arch. Ophthal. **164**, 399—410 (1962).

STRIK, W. O.: Die diagnostische Anwendung des Ultraschalls. Med. Klin. **56,** 1817—1822 (1961).

SUFFCZYŃSKA-KOTOWSKA, A. K., KULESZA, A., MAZUROWA, M.: Obserwacje przypadków fenyloketonurii ze szczególnym uwzglednieniem badań EEG i pneumencefalografii. Ped. Pol. **41,** 1369 (1966).

SUGAR, O., UEMATSU, S.: The use of ultrasound in the diagnosis of intracranial lesions. Surg. Clin. N. Amer. **44,** 55—64 (1964).

SUNDEN, B.: On the diagnostic value of ultrasound in obstetrics and gynaecology. Acta obstet. gynec. scand. **43,** Suppl. 6 (1964).

TAKEUCHI, T.: An experimental study of stereotoxic destruction of cat brain by focused ultrasound. Nihon Geka Hokan **34,** 634—650 (1965).

TANAKA, K.: Diagnosis of brain tumors using ultrasound. Nihon Igaku (Japan. Medic.) Supplementum **III,** 205—209 (1963).

— Diagnosis of brain disease by ultrasound. Shindan-To-Chiryo Sh Co. Ltd. Tokyo 1968.

— ITO, K.: Diagnosis of brain tumor using ultrasound. Acta radiol. (Stockh.) **5,** 915—927 (1966).

— — Ultrasonic diagnosis of intracranial disease. Shinkei Kenkyû no Shimpo (Recent Advances Research Nervous System) **7,** 335—351 (1963).

— — ISHIKAWA, S.: Ultrasonic diagnosis of brain tumor. Sôgô Igaku (Medicine, Tokyo) **18,** 297—308 (1961).

— — — UEMATSU, S.: Cerebral diagnosis in children by means of ultrasound. Shônika Shinryô **25,** 926—932 (1962).

— — — YUKISHITA, K., OHARA, Y.: Ultrasonics in the diagnosis of intracranial space occupying lesions. Proc. III. Intern. Congr. Neurol. Surg., Excerpta medica Intern. Congr. Series **110,** 580—589 (1966).

— — — WAGAI, T.: Diagnosis of brain tumors using ultrasound. Nihon Rinshô (Japan J. clin. Med.) **21,** 2195—2200 (1963).

— — KIKUCHI, Y., UCHIDA, R., UEMATSU, S.: Ultrasonic diagnosis in Japan. In: Diagnostic ultrasound. Eds.: C. C. GROSSMAN et al. New York: Plenum Press 1966, pp. 27—45.

— — OHARA, Y.: Ultrasonotomography of the brain. Intern. Symposium Echo-Encephalographie. Erlangen 14./15. April 1967.

— — WAGAI, T.: The localization of brain tumors by ultrasonic techniques. A clinical review of 111 cases. J. Neurosurg. **23,** 135—147 (1965).

— KIKUCHI, Y., UCHIDA, R.: Detection of intracranial anatomical abnormalities by ultrasound. J. acoust. Soc. Jap. **8**/2, 111—112 (1952).

— — — Ultrasonic diagnosis of brain tumor. Proc. 3rd. int. Congr. Acoust. Stuttgart. Amsterdam: Elsevier Publ. Co. 1959, pp. 1291—1294.

— — — Ultrasonic diagnosis of intracranial diseases. Proc. surg. Soc. Japan **53,** 242—243 (1963).

— WAGAI, T.: Ultrasonic diagnosis of brain disease in Japan. In: Ultrasound as a diagnostic and surgical tool. Ed.: D. GORDON. Edinburg-London: Livingstone 1964, pp. 161—175.

— — ITO, K., UEMATSU, S., ABE, Y., ISHIKAWA, S., KIKUCHI, Y.: Diagnosis of intracranial hemorrhage. In: Advance of medical application of ultrasound developed by the Ultrasonic Research Group in Juntendo University in 1963. Tokyo: Juntendo University School of Medicine, Hongo, 1964.

TANK, T. M., HAMBY, W. B.: Echoencephalography: An aid in the diagnosis of intracranial lesions. Report of a case. Cleveland Clin. Quart. **31,** 101—105 (1964).

TAVERAS, J. M., WOOD, E. H.: Diagnostic neuroradiology. Baltimore: Williams & Williams Co. 1964.

TAYLOR, J. C., NEWELL, J. A., KARVOUNIS, P.: Ultrasonics in the diagnosis of intra-cranial space-occupying lesions. Lancet **1961 I,** 1197—1199.

THEISMANN, H., PFANDER, F.: Über die Durchlässigkeit des Knochens für Ultraschall. Strahlentherapie **80,** 607—610 (1949).

THOMPSON, H. E.: Studies of fetal growth by ultrasound. In: Diagnostic Ultrasound. Eds.: C. C. GROSMAN et al. New York: Plenum Press 1966.

THUN, F.: Die Echoencephalographie bei postoperativen Komplikationen. Acta neurochir. (Wien) **12,** 652 (1965).

TÖNNIS, W.: Die Chirurgie des Gehirns und seiner Häute. Bd. III. In: Die Chirurgie. Hrsg.: M. KIRSCHNER und O. NORDMANN. Wien: Urban & Schwarzenberg 1948.
— Wie läßt sich die Frühdiagnose der Hirntumoren verbessern? Wien. med. Wschr. **103**, 835—840 (1953).
— Diagnostik der intrakraniellen Geschwülste. In: Handbuch der Neurochirurgie. Bd. IV, 3. Teil. Hrsg.: H. OLIVECRONA und W. TÖNNIS. Berlin: Springer 1962.
— BORCK, W. F.: Über Großhirntumoren des Kindesalters. Zbl. Neurochir. **13**, 72—98 (1953).
— FRIEDMANN, G., SCHMITT-WITTKAMP, E., WALTER, W.: Die traumatischen intrakraniellen Hämatome. Documenta Geigy, Series chir. **6**, 1—89 (1963).
— FROWEIN, R. A.: Klinische Fehldiagnosen bei intrakraniellen Hämatomen. Dtsch. Röntgenkongreß 1965. Stuttgart: Thieme 1966, S. 137—142.
— — EULER, K. H.: Zur Erkennung der akuten traumatischen intrakraniellen Haematome. Chirurg **34**, 145—151 (1963).
— LOEW, F., GROTE, W., HEMMER, R., KLUG, W., FINKEMEYER, H.: Organisation der Behandlung schwerer Schädel-Hirn-Verletzungen. Stuttgart: Thieme 1967.
— SCHIEFER, W.: Klinik der raumbeengenden Prozesse des Occipitallappens. Dtsch. Z. Nervenheilk. **170**, 402—432 (1953).
— — Die Komplikationen bei Angiographie der Hirngefäße. Fortschr. Neurol. Psychiat. **26**, 265—300 (1958).
— — Zirkulationsstörungen des Gehirns im Serienangiogramm. Berlin: Springer 1959.
TORKILDSEN, A.: Ventriculo-cisternostomy. A post-operative study. Acta chir. scand. **85**, 254—260 (1941).
— A follow-up study 14 to 20 years after ventriculocisternostomy. Acta psychiat. scand. **35**, 113—121 (1960).
UEMATSU, S.: Ultrasonics determination of the hemispheral thickness for the diagnosis of hydrocephalus. In: Diagnostic Ultrasound. Eds.: C. C. GROSSMAN et al. New York: Plenum Press 1966, pp. 148—154.
— SUGAR, O., WALKER, A. E.: Echoencephalography for head trauma. Amsterdam: Excerpta Medica Foundation 1966.
— — — Echoencephalography for head trauma. Proc. III. Intern. Congr. Neurol. Surg., Excerpta medica Inter. Congr. Series **110**, 194—199 (1966).
— WALKER, A. E.: Ultrasonic determination of the size of cerebral ventricular system. Neurology (Minneap.) **17**, 81—86 (1967).
ULBRICHT, W.: Rückenmarkstumoren mit Stauungspapille. Acta neurochir. **15**, 138—149 (1966).
— DE SEIXAS, V.: Echoencephalographie und 3. Ventrikel. Vortrag Ungar. Neurologenkongreß. Budapest 7.—10. Okt. 1966.
— — Echo-encephalographische Untersuchungen bei Hydrocephali verschiedener Genese, insbesondere beim kindlichen Hydrocephalus. Intern. Symposium Echo-Encephalographie. Erlangen 14./15. April 1967.
UMBACH, W.: Echodiagnostik und Verlaufskontrollen beim kindlichen Hydrocephalus. Acta neurochir. (Wien) **13**, 581 (1965).
— KLEY, M.: Untersuchungen mit Ultraschall zur Diagnose und Verlaufskontrolle des kindlichen Hydrocephalus. Dtsch. med. Wschr. **90**, 1313—1315 (1965).
UNGER, R. R., SIEDSCHLAG, W.-D.: Echoencephalographie und gedeckte Schädel-Hirn-Verletzungen. Mschr. Unfallheilk. **69**, 435—442 (1966).
— — Echoencephalographie und Hirntumor. Dtsch. Gesundh.Wes. **22**, 455—457 (1967).
U.S. Atomic Energy Commission: Studies in methods in instruments to improve localization of radioactive materials in the body with special reference to the diagnosis of brain tumors and the use of ultrasonic techniques. AECU-3012. Minneapolis: Univ. Minnesota Press 1955.
VAN DER DRIFT, J. H. A.: The significance of electro-encephalography for the diagnosis and localization of cerebral tumours. Leiden: H. E. Steifert Kroese N. V. 1957.
VAN DE WEYER, K. H., SAMII, M., SCHURMANN, K.: Beitrag zur Diagnostik ventrikulärer und ventrikelnaher Tumoren mit Hirnstammbeteiligung. Fortschr. Röntgenstr. **III**, 2 (1969).

VIGOUROUX, R. P., FROWEIN, R. A.: Survey of the organization of services for acute head injury in European countries. Amsterdam: Excerpta Medica Foundation 1966.

VINCENT, J. D., FAURE, J., GOT, M., SOUMIREU-MOURAI, B., ESCHAPASSE, P.: Premiers résultats d'utilisation de l'échoencéphalographie en service d'exploration fonctionelle du système nerveux. J. Méd. Bordeaux **143**, 357—365 (1966).

VLIEGER, M. DE: Echo-encephalographie bei Hirnverletzungen. Acta neurochir. (Wien) **9**, 707 (1961).

— Diagnostische hulpmiddelen bij traumatische hersenletsels. Huisarts en Wetenschap **5**, 337—339 (1962).

— Echo-encephalography and extra-cerebral haematomas. In: Ultrasound as a Diagnostic and Surgical Tool. Ed.: D. GORDON. Edinburgh-London: Livingstone 1964, pp. 145—160.

— De mogelijkheden van het twee-dimensionale echogram voor de algemene medische diagnostik. Ned. T. Geneesk. **108**, 1513—1514 (1964).

— Echo-encephalografie en hersendiagnostiek. Hoofdlijnen **1**, 18—23 (1965).

— Ultraschall am geschlossenen Schädel. Schweiz. med. Wschr. **99**, 998—1003 (1969).

— Differentialdiagnostische Schwierigkeiten auf dem Gebiet des Hämatomechos bei posttraumatischen intrakraniellen Blutungen. Intern. Symposium Echo-Encephalographie. Erlangen 14./15. April 1967.

— Die zweidimensionale Echo-Encephalographie beim Hydrocephalus. Intern. Symposium Echo-Encephalographie. Erlangen 14./15. April 1967.

— Echo-Encephalography and cerebral circulation. Excerpta medica, International Congress Series **139**, No. 21 (1967).

— DENIER VAN DER GON, J. J., VAN DER LUGI, P. J. M., MOLIN, C. E.: Pulsations in echoencephalography. 6th Intern. Congr. Electroencephalogr. Clin. Neurophysiol. Wien, Sept. 5—10 1965, pp. 591—592.

— RIDDER, J.: Use of echoencephalography. Neurology (Minneap.) **9**, 216—223 (1959).

— STERKE, A. DE, MOLIN, C. E., VAN DER VEN, C.: Ultrasound for two-dimensional echoencephalography. Ultrasonics **1**, 148—151 (1963).

VOGELSANG, H.: Pneumencephalogramm-Verlaufsbeobachtungen bei Torkildsendrainagen. Deutscher Röntgenkongreß 1964. Stuttgart: Thieme 1965, S. 307—311.

WACHSMANN, F. H.: Schädigungsmöglichkeiten durch Ultraschall vom Standpunkt der physikalischen Vorgänge im Gewebe und der Applikationstechnik aus gesehen. Ultraschall in Med. **4**, 42—44 (1952).

WAGAI, T., MIYAZAWA, R., ITO, K., KIKUCHI, Y.: Ultrasonic diagnosis od intracranial disease, breast tumors and abdominal diseases. In: Ultrasonic Energy. Ed.: E. KELLY. Urbana: University of Illinois Press 1965, pp. 346—364.

— TSUCHIDATE, M., ITO, K., ISHII, M., KATSUMI, S., UEMATSU, S., ISHIKAWA, S., TAKEUHI, T., OHASHI, H., NONOKA, H., TAKEUCHI, K., ABE, Y., ARIMA, M., OUCHI, T., KIKUCHI, Y., IDE, M., UCHIDA, R.: Recent advance of medical application of ultrasound developed by the ultrasonic research group in Juntendo University. Juntendo University School of Medicine, Hongo, Tokyo, Japan 1963.

WAKEFIELD, G.: Ultrasonic diagnosis in cerebral diseases. Univ. Coll. Hosp. Mag. **47**, 10 (1964).

WALKER, A. E., UEMATSU, S.: Dural echoencephalography. J. Neurosurg. **25**, 634—637 (1966).

— HOPPLE, T. L.: Brain tumors in children. J. Pediat. **35**, 671—687 (1949).

WALLACE, W. K., AVANT, W. S., JR., MCKINNEY, W. M., THURSTONE, F.: Ultrasonic techniques for measuring intracranial pulsations. Research and clinical studies. Neurology (Minneap.) **16**, 380—382 (1966).

WATSON, C. W., NIGAM, M. P., PAINE, R. S.: Electroencephalographic abnormalities in phenylpyruvic oligophrenia. Neurology (Minneap). **18**, 203, 1968.

WEBER, R., DILLING, H.: Chirurgie des Gehirns und Rückenmarks im Kindes- und Jugendalter. Hrsg.: K. A. BUCHE und P. GLESS. Stuttgart: Hippokrates, S. 160—169.

WEIGELDT, H. D., SCHRÖTER, K.: Über anatomische und technische Ursachen von echo-encephalographischen Fehlmessungen. Intern. Symposium Echo-Encephalographie. Erlangen 14./15. April 1967.

WEINLAND, W. L., WEINLAND, G.: Erfahrungen mit dem Echo-Encephalogramm in der neurologischen Facharztpraxis. Intern. Symposium Echo-Encephalographie. Erlangen 14./15. April 1967.

WRIGHT, S., TARJAN, G.: Phenylketonuria. Amer. J. Dis. Child. **97**, 405 (1957).

WERTHEIMER, P., FISCHER, G., COURJON, J., GERIN, P., REVOL, M., MUNIER, F.: La valeur diagnostique de l'écho-encéphalographie. Etude d'une statistique de 1000 examens. Rev. Neurol. **114**, 219—225 (1966).

WEST, K. A.: Eko-encefalografi. Suomen Laarkarilehti **19**, 2227—2234 (1964).

— Correlation between ultrasonic and roentgenological findings in infantile hydrocephalus. Acta paed. scand. **56**, 27—36 (1967).

WHITE, N. D.: A-Scan echoencephalography. Canad. Med. Ass. J. **94**, 180—189 (1966).

— Studies in ultrasonic echoencephalography VI. A critical analysis of the amplitude-averaging, A-scan-technique. Neurology (Minneap.) **16**, 858—866 (1966).

— Studies in ultrasonic echoencephalography (6 A). A critical analysis of amplitude averaged A-Scan. Trans. Amer. neurol. Ass. 363—365 (1966).

— Accuracy of A-scan determination of midline echo. In: Diagnostic Ultrasound. Eds.: C. C. GROSSMAN et al. New York: Plenum Press 1966, pp. 142—147.

— The limitations of echoencephalography. Ultrasonics **5**, 88—90 (1967).

— Results of the amplitude-averaged technique of echo-encephalography. 8e Symposium neuroradiol. Paris 1967.

— BLANCHARD, B.: Studies in ultrasonic echoencephalography. IV. Results of an averaging technique to localize the cerebral midline structure. Neurology (Minneap.) **15**, 1041—1048 (1965).

— — Studies in ultrasonic echoencephalography. II. An objective technique for the A-scan presentation of the cerebral midline structures. Acta radiol. 5, diagnosis, 7th Symposium neuroradiol., New York 1964, 936—952 (1966).

— — CLARK, J. M.: Studies in ultrasonic echoencephalography. V. Echoes obtainable from a plastic skull. Brit. J. Radiol. **40**, 108—119 (1967).

— — WHITE, M. N.: Studies in ultrasonic echoencephalography. III. Limitations of a simple radial scan. Wiss. Z. Humboldt-Univ. Berlin, Math.-Nat. R. **14**, 23—28 (1965).

— CHESEBROUGH, J. N., BLANCHARD, J. B.: Studies in ultrasonic echoencephalography. I. A-scan determination of the M-echo position in a group of patients. Neurology (Minneap.) **15**, 81—86 (1965).

— CLARK, J. M., CHESEBROUGH, J. N., WHITE, M. N., CLARK, D. J.: The effect of the skull in degrading resolution in echoencephalographic B- and C-scans. Intern. Symposium Echo-Encephalographie. Erlangen 14./15. April 1967.

— — WHITE, M. N.: Studies in ultrasonic echoencephalography. VII. General principles of recording informations in ultrasonic B- and C-scanning and the effects of scatter, reflection and refraction by cadaver skull on this information. Med. biol. Engng. **5**, 3—14 (1967).

— — — Studies in ultrasonic echoencephalography. VIII. The effects on resolution of irregularities in attenuation of an ultrasonic beam traversing cadaver skull. Med. biol. Engng. **5**, 15—23 (1967).

WIDÉN, L., PERSON, A., WENNBERG, A.: Echo-encephalography in the differential diagnosis between intracerebral haemorrhage and cerebral infraction. Thule Intern. Sympos. Stockholm: Nord. Bokhandelns Förlag 1967, pp. 153—158.

WIEDAU, E., RÖHER, O.: Ultraschall in der Medizin. Dresden-Leipzig: Steinkopff 1963.

WILCKE, O.: Hirntumor-Diagnostik mit Positronenstrahlern. Acta neurochir. (Wien) **10**, 301 bis 319 (1962).

— Möglichkeiten und Grenzen der Hirntumordiagnostik mit Positronenstrahlern (C^{64} und As^{74}). Neurochirurgia **7**, 33—41 (1964).

WILD, J. J.: The use of ultrasonic pulses for the measurement of biologic tissues and the detection of tissue density changes. Surgery **27**, 183—188 (1950).

— REID, J. M.: Application of echo-ranging techniques to the determination of structure of biological tissues. Science **115**, 226—230 (1952).

WILD, J. J., REID, J. M.: Further pilot echographic studies on the histologic structure of tumor of the living intact human breast. Amer. J. Path. **28**, 839—861 (1952).

— — The effects on biological tissues of 15-Mc pulsed ultrasound. J. acoust. Soc. Amer. **25**, 270—280 (1953).

— — Echographic visualization of lesions of the living human breast. Cancer Res. **14**, 277 to 283 (1954).

— — Fifteen megacycle pulsed ultrasonic reflection studies. Ultraschall in Med. **6**, 195—199 (1953).

— — Diagnostic use of ultrasound. Brit. J. Phys. Med. **19**, 248—257 (1956).

WILLARD, G. W.: Improved methods for measuring ultrasonic velocity. J. acoust. Soc. Amer. **23**, 83—93 (1951).

WILLICH, E., MOSTAFAWY, A.: Die Dyostosis pelvico-cleido-cranialis. Fortschritte auf dem Gebiet der Röntgenstrahlen und der Nuklearmedizin **113**, 49—59 (1970).

WILLOCKS, J., DONALD, I., DUGGAN, T. C., DAY, N.: Foetal cephalometry by ultrasound. J. Obstet. Gynaec. Brit. Cwlth. **71**, 11—20 (1964).

— The use of ultrasonic cephalometry. Proc. roy. Soc. Med. **55**, 640 (1962).

WOEBER, K. H.: Über das Auftreten von Schädigungen am Zentralnervensystem der Ratte durch Ultraschallwellen. Strahlentherapie **79**, 643—652 (1949).

WOOD, R. W., LOOMIS, A. L.: Physical and biological effects of high-frequency sound-waves of great intensity. Phys. Rev. **29**, 373 (1927), zit. nach L. BERGMANN.

YAMAKAWA, K., YOSHIOKA, A.: Ultrasonic diagnostic methods. Sôgô Igaku (Medicine, Tokyo) **20**, 265—271 (1963).

YANG, C. L., and TAN, Y. L.: Ultrasonic examination of 170 patients with intracranial hypertension. (Zhongua Shenjingjingshnke Zazhi.) Science abstracts China Medicine **5**, 26 (1964).

YUKISHITA, K.: Ultrasonic diagnosis of brain tumor. Arch. jap. chir. **37**, 234—160 (1968).

— ABE, Y., ITO, K., WAGAI, T.: Ultrasonics in the diagnosis of head injury. Japan. Med. Ultrasonics **3**, 29 (1965).

— EHARA, K., NONAKA, H., ISHIKAWA, S., ITO, K., TANAKA, K.: Ultrasonics in the diagnosis of brain tumor [3rd report. Med. Ultrasonics **4**, 59 (1966)].

— TANAKA, K., ITO, K.: Ultrasonic diagnosis of brain tumors. Intern. Symposium Echo-Encephalographie. Erlangen 14./15. April 1967.

ZANDER, E., FOROGLOU, G.: L'apport de l'échoencephalographie en neurochirurgie. Praxis **55**, 398—406 (1966).

ZICHNER, L.: Zur Bedeutung der Echoencephalographie in der klinischen Neurologie. Inaug.-Diss. Düsseldorf 1967.

ZÜLCH, K. J.: Die Hirngeschwülste in biologischer und morphologischer Darstellung. 3. Auflage. Leipzig: J. Abrosius Barth 1958.

— Morphologische Voraussetzungen für das abnorme Echo-Encephalogramm. Intern. Symposium Echo-Encephalographie. Erlangen 14./15. April 1967.

— FISCHGOLD, ED.: L'électrencéphalographie dans les déplacements en masse du cerveau. 9e réunion européenne d'information électroencéphalographique. Marseille 12./13. Oct. 1960.

Subject Index

A-form echo 48
A-scope technique 7, 12, 16
Abscess, cerebral 52, 102, 103, 104
—, —, illustrative case 101
Acoustical interface 4, 5, 6, 9, 10, 13, 83
— impedance 4, 5, 6, 19
— —, of tumor tissue 49
Adenoma, echo form 49
Amplification 10
Amplifier 9
Angiogram, carotid 87, 95, 100, 104, 105
Arc scanning 12, 13, 16
Astrocytoma 49, 95, 96, 107, 108
— echo 50, 108
—, illustrative cases 95, 107

B-scan technique 16
B-scope technique 7, 16
Bottom echo 17
Brain mantle index 24, 26, 30, 34
— — —, calculation of 26, 34
— — —, capability of measurement 24, 26, 27
— — —, comparison to LVI 27
— — —, erroneous measurement of 85
— — —, hydrocephalus and 45
— — —, normal values 27, 35
— — —, PEG-SEG studies of 35
— — thickness 45, 46
— — —, measurement of 80
— — —, reaction to pressure alleviation 80
— trauma (see Trauma) 36 ff.

C-scope technique 7
Callipers 14
Cathode ray tube 7, 10, 12
Cella media 74 ff., 85, 86
Cerebral atrophy 18, 30, 87, 97, 98, 101, 102
— —, EEG findings and 90, 97, 101
— —, illustrative cases 97, 99
— —, intelligence in 64
— —, midline echo in 30, 91, 92, 97
— —, PEG in 102
— —, phenylketonuria and 58 ff.
— —, SEG findings 30, 55, 57, 91, 102
— calcifications 28

Cerebral death 19
— edema, post-traumatic 36
— —, in tumors 51
— falx, as source of error 84
— palsy 54
Compound scanning 12, 13, 16
Concussion, cerebral 36 ff.
Congenital defects 30, 54 ff.
Congenital defects, midline echo in 30
— —, SEG findings 55, 57
— —, vascular 87
Contusion, cerebral 36 ff.
—, midline shift in 36
—, ventricular dilation in 36
Convulsive disorders 64 ff.
— —, PEG in 65
— —, SEG findings in 64, 65
Coupling 12
Cranial circumference 30, 81
— —, comparison with SEG results 69
— diameter 15, 74
— —, calculation of 18, 23
Craniopharyngioma, echo pattern in 49, 50
Cystic wall echoes 55
Cysts, as source of error 84
—, in cavum vergae 85
—, — septum pellucidum 85

Dandy Walker syndrome 56, 57
Decibel 3
Developmental defects 54 ff.
— —, SEG findings 55, 57, 69
Diaphany 68, 79
Dura echo 39
— mater 9
— —, in epidural hematoma 37

Echo-EG 16
Echoencephalography 16
Effusion echo 40
Electroencephalogram, combined EEG-SEG exam 39, 54, 87 ff.
—, infratentorial mass and 90, 93, 94
—, supratentorial mass and 90, 93, 95
—, in tumors 87 ff., 95, 99, 106, 107
End echo 17, 21, 22, 23
— —, determination 17
— —, in cephalic hematoma 36

Ependymoma 98, 99, 104
—, echo form 49, 50
—, illustrative cases 99, 103
Epilepsy 64, 65, 93
—, SEG in 65
Error sources in SEG 83 ff.
— —, summary of 84
Examination position 13 ff., 85, 88, 89
— procedure, sitting 16
— —, supine 13, 14

Far-side echo 17
Fechner Weber Law 3

Glioblastoma 28
Guthrie test 58, 59

Hearing threshold 3
Hematocephalus 40
Hematoma 36 ff.
—, acute subdural 38
—, — —, SEG findings 39
—, — —, vs epidural 38
—, chronic subdural 39
— echoes 38, 42, 45
— —, examination procedure 38
—, epidural 36, 37
—, —, cause of 37
—, —, echoes in 38
—, —, vs acute subdural 38
—, intracerebral 40, 42, 45
—, —, EEG findings 43
—, —, illustrative cases 41 ff.
—, —, SEG findings 41, 42, 44
—, intracranial 37
—, —, birth-traumatic 81
—, measurement of 38
—, scalp 85
—, subdural 36
—, —, echoes in 38
High frequency oscillator 8
Hydrocephalus 30, 45 ff., 66 ff.
—, brain mantle thickness in 68
—, — tumors and 93, 100, 104
—, clinical findings and 69, 70, 71, 72
—, follow-up studies 78 ff.
—, increased pressure 69, 70, 71
—, infratentorial masses and 53, 92
—, internal 46, 82
—, macrocephalus in 69
—, midline echo in 30
—, occlusive 104
—, pelvico-cleidocranialis dysostosis and 81, 82, 83
—, progressive 69, 70, 71, 79
—, reliability of SEG in 66 ff.
—, supratentorial masses and 53, 92

Hygroma 36 ff.
—, subdural 84
—, —, SEG findings 40

Indicator gauge 10
Infantile encephalopathy 55
Infratentorial lesion, EEG findings 90
— —, SEG findings 28, 53, 91, 105
Initial echo 17, 21, 22, 23
— complex 17
Insula Echoes 25

Jacksonian seizures 97

Laplace's Equation 2
Lateral echoes 25
— ventricles, anatomical form 85
— —, as source of error 84
— —, evaluation of 78
— —, external examination point 15, 21, 67
— —, PEG-SEG comparison 66 ff., 73, 74, 75, 76
— —, posttraumatic dilation of 36
— ventricular echoes 15, 21 ff., 30, 88
— — —, capability of measurement 24, 31
— — —, external examination point 21, 15, 22, 30, 31, 88
— — index, abnormal values 25, 68
— — —, advantage of 73
— — —, calculation of 74
— — —, cerebral atrophy and 55
— — —, classification of 30
— — —, capability of measurement 24, 27
— — —, comparison to BMI 27
— — —, determination of 21, 22 ff., 30, 88
— — —, erroneous measurement of 85
— — —, hydrocephalus and 45
— — —, normal values 25
— — —, pathological 30
— — —, PEG-SEG comparison 77
— — —, phenylketonuria and 59, 62
— — —, in roentgenology 77
Limitations of SEG 83
Linear scanning 12, 13

M-form echo 48
Magnification of film 68
Main bang 17
Medulloblastoma, echo form 49
Meningoma, echo form 49
Midline echo 17, 18, 19, 28, 29, 30, 88
— —, abnormal 29, 88
— —, erroneous measurement of 85
— —, external reference point 67
— —, from falx cerebri 18, 29
— —, — interhemispheric space 18, 29
— —, — pineal body 29

Midline echo, from septum pellucidum 18, 22, 29, 67
— —, origin 18, 22, 29, 67
— —, post-traumatic dilation of 36
— —, pulsation of 19, 29
— —, recognition 29
— —, reliability of 66
— —, sources of error 29, 30, 85
— —, theoretical 15, 18, 30, 88
— shift 28 ff., 88
— —, calculation of 18, 28, 29
— —, cause 28
— —, cerebral atrophy and 55, 91, 92, 93
— —, EEG foci and 88
— —, hematoma and 36, 37, 39, 41
Midline shift, infratentorial masses and 91, 94
— —, normal 18, 29
— —, significant 29, 88
— —, supratentorial masses and 91
— —, tumors and 91
— —, unauthentic 29, 84, 85

Near-side echo 17
Neurinoma echo 49, 50
Nucleus lentiformis 25

Oligodendroglioma 28
—, echo form 49
Osseous cranium, density 29
Oscillator, ceramic 8
— —, sound reflection from 9
— —, thickness of 7, 17, 18, 22, 23, 31, 88

Pachymeningitis internal, hemorrhagic 39
Pachymeningosis serosa 39
Pelvicocleidocranialis dysostosis 81, 82, 83
Phenylketonuria 58 ff.
—, intelligence in 60, 61, 63, 64
—, lateral ventricles in 59, 62
—, morphological findings in 58
—, PEG in 58
—, third ventricle in 59, 62
Phlegmona 85
Phon 3
Piezoelectric crystal 4, 8, 9
Pinal body 29
Pneumoencephalogram, cerebral atrophy and 102
—, — mass and 100, 102, 105
—, comparison with SEG 25, 26, 32, 46
—, Phenylketonuria and 58
Pneumoencephalographic index 32, 74
Porencephaly 55, 79
Pulse intensity 17, 29

Resolving power 8, 9

Saw-tooth voltage 10
Scalp 9
Scan 16
Scope 16
Sector scanning 12, 13, 16
Seizures, in phenylketonuria 62, 64
—, SEG in 64, 65
Septum pellucidum 15
— —, as source of error 84, 85
Skull, diameter of 14
—, measurement of 14
Snell's Law 4
Sonoencephalogram, abnormal 28 ff.
—, combined with angiogram 100, 104, 105
—, — — EEG 87 ff.
—, — — PEG 23, 56, 67, 100, 102, 105
—, normal 17 ff.
Sonoencephalography, special 36 ff.
—, general 1 ff.
Sonogram 10, 11
Sonography 16
Sono-opthalmology 7, 8, 12
Sonotomography 16
Sonoventriculogram 15, 22, 89
Sound, absorption 6, 7, 9, 10
—, attenuation 6
—, classification of 4
—, intensity 3, 4, 5, 7, 9, 10, 29
—, propagation 4, 6, 11
—, probe 8 (see Transducer)
—, reflection 4, 5
— —, conditions favorable to 5
— refraction 4
— scattering 6, 9
— volume 3
— waves 2 ff.
— —, classification 4
— —, definition 2
— —, frequency 2, 4, 10
— —, in gases 3
— —, in liquids 3
— —, in solids 3
— —, length 2, 6
— —, mechanical 2
— —, propagation velocity 2, 4
— —, transverse 2
Space-occupying lesion 18, 48 ff., 87 ff.
— —, EEG alterations 87
— —, illustrative cases 94 ff.
— —, in midline 30, 31
— —, — temporal lobe 30
— —, indirect documentation 28, 48, 51
— —, infratentorial 28, 52, 53, 90 ff.
— —, SEG findings 48, 51, 52, 53
— —, supra vs infratentorial 28, 52, 53, 87 ff.
— —, supratentorial 28, 51, 53, 90 ff.

Space-occupying lesion, value of SEG 48
Spitz-Holter valve 80
Subdural hygroma 69
Subsonic sounds 4
Supratentorial lesion, EEG findings 90, 99, 106, 107
— —, SEG findings 28, 91, 96, 100, 106, 108
Sweep generator 7, 10
Synchronization unit 10

Temporal bone, irregularities 29
— horn, as source of error 84
— — echoes 22, 23, 25, 26
— — —, beam direction 35
— — —, examination procedure 26, 34
— — —, origin of 26
— — —, recognition of 26
Terminology 16
Third ventricle, anatomical shape 20, 34
— —, dilatation 20, 30, 33
— —, erroneous measurement of 85
— —, external examination point 15, 19, 67, 89
— —, hydrocephalus and 45
— —, PEG-SEG comparison 66, 72, 73
— —, phenylketonuria and 59, 62
— —, post-traumatic dilation of 36
Third ventricle, tumor within 30, 31
— —, as source of error 84
— —, cerebral atrophy and 55, 91
— —, combined PEG-SEG 33, 34
— —, width 19, 20, 30, 32, 33, 89
— ventricular reflections 19, 67
— — —, identification of 20, 33, 32, 89
— — —, origin of 20
— — —, pulsation of 32
Transducer (sound probe) 5, 7, 12, 29
Transducer as receiver 9
— as transmitter 8
Transillumination 68, 79
Trauma, brain 36 ff.
—, —, edema in 36
—, —, midline shift in 36
—, —, ventricular dilation in 36
Tumor complex 31
— —, classification of 49
— reflections 48 ff.
— —, A-form echo 48, 49
— —, classification of 49
— —, cystic tumor echo 50
Tumor-reflections, M-form echo 48
— —, physical characteristics of 48
Two-dimensional SEG 7, 10, 12, 16

Ultrasonic attenuation 48
Ultrasound, apparatus 7 ff.
—, A-scope 7, 16
—, B-scan 16
—, B-scope 16
—, definition 4
—, in cardiology 16
—, — internal medicine 7, 16
—, — obstetrics and gynecology 7, 8
—, — surgery 7
—, physical characteristics of 4
— receiver 7, 9
—, transmitter 7, 8, 9
Unidimensional SEG 7, 10, 16

Wall echoes, cystic 55
Water path scanning 16
Wehyelt cylinder 12

X-ray divergence 34, 72, 73

MIX
Papier aus verantwortungsvollen Quellen
Paper from responsible sources
FSC® C105338

If you have any concerns about our products,
you can contact us on
ProductSafety@springernature.com

In case Publisher is established outside the EU,
the EU authorized representative is:
Springer Nature Customer Service Center GmbH
Europaplatz 3, 69115 Heidelberg, Germany

Printed by Libri Plureos GmbH
in Hamburg, Germany